PSYCHE

and family

PSYCHE
and family

Jungian Applications to Family Therapy

edited by
Laura S. Dodson & Terrill L. Gibson

Chiron Publications ■ *Asheville, North Carolilla*

Library of Congress Catalog Card Number: 96–xxxxx

Printed in the United States of America.
Copyedited by Andrew C. Baker.
Book design by Siobhan Drummond.
Cover design by D.J. Hyde.

Library of Congress Cataloging-in-Publication Data:

Psyche and family : Jungian applications to family therapy / Laura S. Dodson and Terrill L. Gibson, editors
p. cm—(Psyche and world series)
Includes bibliographical references
1. Family psychotherapy. 2. Jungian psychology. I. Dodson, Laura Sue. I. Gibson, Terill L., 1946– . III. Series
RC488.5.P766 1996
616.89'156—dc20 96-25236
CIP

ISBN 978—1—63051—541—6 (pbk.)

CONTENTS

DEDICATION AND ACKNOWLEDGMENTS

This book is the outgrowth of life with parents and siblings, and of my relationship with my husband, George, and my children, Jon and Corina. I thank them all for being a theater of learning for my life, with highs and lows, with positive intent, and with love. I wish to thank my clients, who are my constant teachers. Professionally, Virginia Satir was my primary teacher, colleague, and friend for twenty-four years before her death in 1988. She added dynamite and humor to my training and analysis in Freudian work. In her later years we shared systems work internationally, and worked toward expanding family systems thought to the world as a system.

A teacher of profound significance for me was James Hall, with whom I interned after studying at the Jung Institute in Zurich during 1972–73. I came to Jung from an immersion in Freudian psychoanalysis and in family systems practice and theory, psychodrama and group therapy. James Hall helped me to integrate Jung and systems. Jungians with similar passions, like Marian Woodman, have inspired me along the way as well. My dear Russian and Eastern European colleagues—for whom system, spirituality and culture *are* psychology—have inspired me and contributed greatly to my practice, my family, and my life.

It is to these friends, family, clients, and colleagues that I dedicate this work. Thank you for your investment in me.

Laura Dodson

Life is alchemy and family is its krater. And I had all my families gathered about me as I assembled this collection with Laura. I am grateful for my ancestors in Kansas, Kentucky, Scotland, Prussia, and the Cherokee Nation. I heard their farmer, hunter, medicine, poet, weaver, and musician voices between every line of this text. I am learning more and more to see the hidden blessings in all that my family of origin and I struggled to say and see across all these years of co-living and co-suffering.

I am moved, often beyond image and word, by the rich and extensive family of mentors and colleagues who helped knead my professional soul over the decades, especially John Allan, Jim Aylward, Doug Anderson, Harrell Beck, Louise Bode, Pamela

Burdick, Will Dixon, Katherine Dyckman, Barbara Fisher, Gene Harvey, Jud Howard, Pat Hudson, Jim Ingersoll, Homer Jernigan, Merle Jordan, Neal Kuyper, Russ Lockhart, Penny Matthews, Wayne McCleskey, Mary Mulig, Mel Ritchey, Don Smith, Duane Spiers, Orlo Strunk, Bob Stuckey, and many others. My work family keeps a systems view alive for me—my "brother" Jerry Smith, Ted Brackman, and Bob Houk.

My professional colleagues in the American Association of Pastoral Counselors, Northwest Pastoral Counseling, and Jungian Analysts-North Pacific are central soul families for me. Charles Chipps and my Lakota Sioux "family" have been invaluable in reminding me of the still living tribal roots of everyone on the planet.

And a special gratitude for those who so bravely shared and bared their family psyche to me across these now many therapeutic years. And for my life partner, Rosa Beth, who dreams new visions of family by my side every night. And a special hug for all the children who keep my spirit renewed, for my goddaughters and godsons, my nieces and nephew. Thank you, thank you all—you are the living footnotes and bibliography to this book.

Terry Gibson

Introduction

Laura Dodson
and Terrill Gibson

There are always revolutions and revelations in psychotherapy. Such is the instinctual way of a dynamic discipline. But these revolutions and revelations always expose themselves as simply rediscoveries of ancient processes forged and then forgotten.

At first blush, it seems an unlikely revolution to mate family therapy and Jungian analysis—both conceptually and developmentally. Both disciplines have recently been strutting their youthful, independent stuff. Though not a youngster measured in years, Jungian analysis has only recently claimed a more public prestige and respect after years of being the embarrassing, mystical secret in the analytic family closet. Jungian analysis is feeling its oats, and wants its rightful place in the Academy. In many ways, Jungian analysis wants the adolescence and public recognition denied it for too many years.

Family therapy, too, often blows its own horn of proud, youthful self-reliance and completeness. It often believes it is a totally new systems look at the world, an earth-shaking "paradigm-shift" that needs to divorce itself from its analytic parents, and their hoary ideas from an outdated clinical past.

But it is the developmental and conceptual vigor in each discipline that makes attractive the idea of mating their energies and vision. Both offer sweeping and inclusive views of the clinical terrain that invite wide interdisciplinary speculation and dialogue. Both respect and even demand a world-view that gets well beyond the skin of an exclusively intrapsychic treatment economy. For the Jungian, there is a vast collective unconscious, an Objective Psyche, beyond the garden wall of the personal unconscious. For the family therapist, there is a vast interlocking web of being and meaning beyond the hub of the individual bonds of the nuclear family. For both models, psyche extends in an infinite number of interpenetrative directions in ways that are both linear and simultaneous. Both systems love this ambiguity and look to such odd companions as modern physicists, totemic ancestors, and biologists with whom to explore findings and wonderings. And both disciplines are increasingly humbled by recognizing that what they once thought revolutionary in their efforts is really but the most recent improvisation on ancient themes of healing myth and culture.

We intend this book to be of broad interest to both consumers and practitioners of the art of psychotherapy. We nurture a special wish that the depth therapist and the marriage and family therapist come to recognize the common passion they share for the unique individuation process which can only occur in some of its dimensions in relationship. For a long period, depth psychotherapies followed the lead of their founding father Freud and focused on a protracted analysis of intra-psychic economies, the outer world suffering a pronounced theoretical impoverishment in analytic writings. For a time, the field of family therapy moved solely in the direction of a strategic and structural deployment of technological interventions within the family system, the inner world of individual experience within the family system suffering a severe theoretical and practice neglect.

But then a great leap of connection sprung up between these two isolates, in the blossoming of object relational work that originally took root in Britain in the 1940s. Analysts seized on object relations for innovative and often breathtaking clinical adaptations of their psychologies of the self in the 1970s, '80s and '90s. At the same time system therapists embraced projective identification notions from object relational psychology, emphasizing the amplifying mirrors between inner and outer image and behavior.

Both fields now stand poised before a rich open landscape of possible collaboration and mutual clinical reinvigoration. Whole new common trends and trajectories are unfolding in a clinical world increasingly focused on holistic thought. Both fields are integrating spirituality into daily praxis, both are impacted by chaos and relativity thinkers, and both are recognizing the centrality of finding and allying with the essence of the change process itself. Both movements find it increasingly easy to reimagine clinical enactment that attempts to recover "the world as a total system" (Boulding 1985).

We are living at the beginning of an exciting post-bias era. This is a pregnant time in history for the multi-geographical and multi-theoretical professions of psychology. Disciplinary zealotry is being exchanged for cross-disciplinary wonder and openness. Eastern European nations, which developed a psychology in isolation from the proud individualism of Freud, are challenging the West with integrations that are at once more communal and mystical. The fall of the Berlin Wall, the failed coup in Russia, and the open struggle with cultural identity in Bosnia challenge us to a global psychology that moves beyond individual growth to systems change on all levels.

The Georgetown family therapy movement, pioneered by Murray Bowen, has a profound and growing interest in the contribution of the natural and evolutionary sciences to the psychotherapy project. The work of Virginia Satir, with its significant contributions about family systems, broadened the dialogue to include spiritual psychology and cultural systems. The Wesley College programs at the Stone Center are bursting the relational seams of conventional depth psychology world views. The lightning of change is striking the ground of practice all around us.

At second glance, this mating of family therapy and Jungian analysis is not so strange at all. This book encourages these two youthful systems to dance together awhile across these pages, to share an event of dialogue and to see what new associations, recognitions, and creations might enrich their combined method and missions. The best things, from good marriages to world peace, often come from such vigorous, relaxed, and eros-tinged encounters. Psychotherapy is, after all, about creating perpetual, healing revolutions, working with the psyche wherever it appears—in a dream or in the family.

This book tries to ease into these lively waters with a simple, focused, and mildly provocative series of essays which suggests something of the revolutionary sweep of these conceptual changes. The two editors, Laura Dodson and Terry Gibson, lead off with descriptions of the ways they have attempted to stretch the individual analytic container to let in the marriage, the family, and the systemic world. Both have had in-depth systemic and analytic training and have struggled for decades to keep their feet in the two world views. They have a deep respect for the developmental, object relational, and intergenerational thinkers who pioneered the way, making such a dialogue possible.

With the door opened by the Dodson and Gibson essays, in walks the couple. Polly Eisendrath-Young meets them head-on with a dialogue therapy rich in both archetypal nuance and strategic common sense. Polly is one of the groundbreakers in this systems-depth conversation, having published her classic reflections on Jungian couple work, *Hags and Heroes* (1984), more than a decade ago.

Murray Stein provocatively reflects on the mythic depth and painful enigma of the sibling bond and bind within the family of origin. Murray has long been interested in the ancient mythic voices and their ongoing augury alive within the contemporary marital and family krater.

While Murray stirs up the sibling pot, Sue Crommelin-Dell unleashes the fascinating fury of adolescent *angst* in her work. Her decades-long exposure to the archetypal depth and nuance of the adolescent process of transitional individuation receives a crisp and vivid telling in an innovative, integrative essay.

Ann Ulanov is one of the best Jungian analytic enunciators and clarifiers of the object relational relevance for the Jungian project. Her subtle narrative gift of precise analysis in her extensive writings comes again to the fore in her satisfying essay on the inner and outer depth alchemy of relationship.

Finally, Renos Papadopoulos brings to full heat Papadopoulos' own systems-archetypal integrative career, a career that has spanned three continents and three decades. Papadopoulos' vigorous and provoking essay on systemic challenges to archetypal work in current context brings this collection of beginning integrative essays to a close. And it is just that, a beginning, but we trust an enticing and productive one for our practicing colleagues who are constantly seeking, as we are, the wider vessel within which to hold the constantly emerging and ever-so-fragile healing truths of our shared work and vision.

References

Boulding, K. 1985. *The World as Total System.* Beverly Hills: Sage Publications.

Young-Eisendrath, P. 1984. *Hags and Heroes: A Feminist Approach to Jungian Psychotherapy with Couples.* Toronto: Inner City Books.

Incest and Imagination

Intergenerational Family Crisis and Transformation in Jungian Analysis

Terrill L. Gibson, Ph.D.

The family is the purest vessel of our destiny. More than the *temenos* of analysis, the sacraments of religion, the most transcendent of experiences, it is family that births us, develops us, procreates us, and buries us. We can never be more or less to life than what has been bequeathed to us by our ancestors. Regardless of the pain and travail it may create for us, family is the grail within which the sacred nectar of our physical and psychic DNA is carried from the lips and genitals of one generation to the next.

With family being so essential, it is puzzling to note its near absence from our analytical literature and practice. Most of the brief citations for family in the index to Jung's *Collected Works* are metaphorical or allegorical. Beyond the occasional work of Eleanor Bertine (1992), Laura Dodson (1983), Adolf Guggenbühl-Craig (1986), Soren Ekstrom (1988), Renos Papadopoulos (1989–90), Hal Stone (1989), or Polly Young-Eisendrath (1984), little of any real analytical or archetypal depth has been written on this important theme. The biological family, the physical manifestations of family, the family of sweat and egg and sperm and tears, is a ghostlike specter in our tradition.

This paper presents a two-part discussion of this dilemma and its implications for our practice. First, some tentative avenues for a renewing integration of family process within analysis are offered, as well as reflections on some of the avoidances and prejudices which have prevented this integration. The central importance of the family incest drama (as a positive, mythic force of development and not just a literal, criminal evil) will be explored. Secondly, some of the possible modifications and examples of technique which might result from such a theoretical *coniunctio* are suggested.

The Family as the Essential Psychospiritual Initiatory Vessel

> *When we tell stories about the family without judgment and without instant analysis . . . family history is transformed into myth. Whether we know it or not, our ideas about the family are rooted in the ways we imagine the family. That personal family, which seems so concrete, is always an imaginal entity. Part of our alchemical work with soul is to extract myth from the hard details of family history and memory on the principle that increase of imagination is always increase in soul.*
>
> —*Moore 1992, 32*

The family is where the imagination seeds. It is the environmental release mechanism for the activation and unfolding of the imaginal soul within us at birth. The hovering, brooding, incessant nurturing of the bio-archetypal Mother and Father validates not only the body and its awakening *sensorium* but also, much more profoundly, the psyche and its awakening spirit-eros. The mediation of the family helps us see not just the phenomenal outer world, but the noumenal inner world as well.

The central theme of this essay is that the primary imaginal lens of psychic development stimulated by this family process is the incest dynamic. Incest is an unavoidable imaginal instigator of soul-process in the human psyche. In order not only to live but to thrive, the psyche must desire life. It must yearn and even suffer after this life, for suffering is the most potent chemical catalyst of desire—the desire for personalized meaning and connection and place in this world. Desire is awakened by the gleam in the Other's Mothering/Fathering Eye. That gleam, and its interpenetrative arousal of our primary soul-self, is our first sexual experience, our first orgasm of total, embodied personhood (Lacan 1977). It is an experience of complete, holistic orgasm where the mystery of being both fully in this world and yet transcendentally assured of a continuity of being beyond this world is mediated. It is a moment primordially incestuous—for the desire is complete and all-consuming for both beloved infant and the beloving Other.

But it must be a developmentally appropriate and healthy

incest which is mediated. Such an incest can differentiate between imaginal and literal incest. Only a parent who has been well and appropriately beloved in childhood can so love appropriately in adulthood. Such a parent has no need for the infant to hold him as beloved. Such a parent does not need to literalize her love for her child. They can live in the incest-driven symbiosis of mutual attraction, willing to absorb the devouring of the physical and emotional feeding of the infant. They can incorporate these often envious infant gluttonies, and can lovingly, empathically guide the child without fear or anger. They are so aware of an autonomous, fully alive, independent infant self that they can gently make this incestuous sacrifice without reactivity or rancor.

This essay advocates the inherent necessity and creativity of this psychological incest process. It sees psychotherapy and analysis as the alchemical krater in which to re-arouse slumbering incestuous dragons and to reinvoke their healing possibilities.

Family as Initiatory *Temenos*: Finding a Safe, Aesthetic Place for Redemptive Suffering

> *Certainly the world is immeasurably beautiful,*
> *but it is also quite as horrible.*
>
> *—Jung 1963, 58*

Analytical psychology is so diverse that generalizations about our commonly held presuppositions are increasingly difficult (Samuels 1985; Stein 1982). But all the varying factions of practice seem to hold a central commitment to the importance of the container of therapy, the *temenos*, the *vas bene secum*. That the psyche must feel safely "held" (most often but not necessarily a long-term process) by a trusted guardian seems indisputable. I know of no intentionally brief therapists among Jungians. The long-term provision, securing, and holding of the therapeutic frame seems a universally axial standard of practice in our ranks. The *how* of that technology may be in dispute, but not its centrality.

In the natural world, two such organically occurring containers exist—the archetypal family and connection to the biological Self. Analysis exists not to transplant these vessels but to enhance their presence. In a dualist culture, such an artificial invention as analysis seems to be a necessary measure to assure memory of and competent access to both these ancient thresholds of psychic maturation.

Analytical and archetypal psychologies make an undisputed contribution to the engagement of the first of these thresholds. Though our appreciation for, description of, and utilization of the treasures of the archetypal Self may be lively debated (Hall and Young-Eisendrath 1988), its manifest and animated presence in our lives and work is incontrovertible.

Why, then, this puzzling absence of recognition of, or even reference to, family in our work? Why the troubling lack of family involvement and resource? The psyche is inherently tribal. The vast corpus of the cross-cultural investigations of, for example, Campbell (1988) or Eliade (1978) makes this clear. The family first receives the archetypal projections of the emergent Self. The family is the necessary catalyst for the developmental appearance, sequencing, and empowering of these archetypal media both biologically and psychospiritually. To do analysis without the family, then, seems a bit like attempting to blow glass without fire. The gestures and procedures may all be precise, but the annealing catalyst of the process is absent.

Of course, the family presence is pervasive in the analytical process. Patients dream of their families' interactions, reactions, and abreactions to their analytical process every night. Murray Bowen, a psychoanalytically trained pioneer of modern family therapies, often saw individuals alone—profoundly aware, at the same time, that he was always doing family therapy (Bowen 1981). The family—the whole family, including all of the ancestors—is always in our offices in every moment of analytic exchange. We cannot escape family and its influence in our practice. Family broods over us from conception until death; family midwives the soul; family makes or breaks an analytical endeavor. We have no choice in involving or excluding the family in our therapies. As with all else in our work, we can only chose to receive and interact with family consciously or unconsciously.

Jungian psychology at its best and worst is a theatrical psychology. It is a psychology with a public nimbus around its head, a therapy of perceived pizzazz and panache. It is a therapy of the Big Event, the Big Dream, the theophanies of the archetypal world. Sadly, it is also a therapy usually reserved for the culturally and materially elite because of its often ominous price tag.

This image is unfortunate and destructive. I want a Jungian

psychology of the marketplace, of the everyday. I want an archetypal world without fancy packaging and marketing. I want dreams of bowels and flesh—psychic encounters in the vernacular. If this everyday is not addressed, it will consume us and destroy us, for the everyday is the most potent container of psyche's essence:

> Every time we try to deal with our outrage over the freeway, our misery over the office and the lighting and the crappy furniture, the crime on the streets, whatever—every time we try to deal with that by going to therapy with our rage and fear, we're depriving the political world of something. And therapy, in its crazy way, by emphasizing the inner soul and ignoring the outer soul, supports the decline of the actual world. (Hillman 1992, 5)

This "real" world is home to Hillman's *anima mundi*—the imaginal realm where real world spirit regains its zest and vision. The real world must be addressed and embraced at the core of therapy's ponderings and sufferings after transformation. In the everyday, the best of the "unfathomable, multiple, prior, generative . . . highly intentional and necessary" archetypal world of both the "noumenal" and the "phenomenal" manifests itself (Moore 1992, 25–32; Hillman 1992, 13). And the best of the everyday is our tribal, familial context.

The Ego-Self-Other Axis: In the Psyche, All Roads Lead Back Home

> *We bring the dysfunctions of family into the therapy room as problems to be solved or as explanations for current difficulties because intuitively we know that the family is one of the chief abodes of the soul . . . . If we were to observe the soul in the family by honoring its stories and by not running away from its shadow, then we might not feel so inescapably determined by family influences . . . . [A] renewed entry into the family, embracing what has previously been denied, often leads to an unexpected alchemy in which even the most difficult family relationships shift enough to make*

> *a significant difference . . . . Family history is transformed into myth.*
>
> —*Moore 1992, 25–32*

The ego-Self axis construct has become one of the favorite theoretical shorthands for Jungians in recent years (Edinger 1972, 73). Along with the complex, the opposites, and individuation itself, the ego-Self axis construct has become a significant organizing cluster of considerable power, with all sorts of conscious and unconscious associations. Connotations of development, of depth, of integration, of upper and lower—much of the best of Jung's original vision into the prospective functions of the psyche—are amply and respectfully echoed in this felicitous concept. It has become a term both conceptually rich and methodologically useful.

But it lacks breadth. The metaphor insinuates and explores the vertical, physio-spatial dimensions of top-to-bottom, heaven-to-earth, psyche-to-soma. But it excludes the horizontal aspects of our companionate, communal, earthly existence. It precludes reference to the tribe, the family, the everyday. It extends the Jungian (and often elitist and solipsistic) metaphor of the individual mining the infinite resources of his her/his own psychic ore shaft, alone, in the pure uncontaminated wilderness of the individuating quest.

Where is the Other in this paradigm—both the everyday relational other and the extraordinary, but *relationally* beloved Divine Other? I suggest expanding the metaphor to a trinitarian ego-Self-Other image. For psychic work really demands a covenant with all three corners of the pyramid of psyche—the ego, the Self, and the Other. All are animated, sentient, contracting partners in the covenantal dialogue and commitment to the individuating project. All three have a profound investment in the outcome of the conversation and contracting an outcome which affects the future health and development of each.

Family is the most prominent landmark on the horizontal plane of relational otherness. Family mediates this world and its essential, phenomenal reality for both the ego and the Self. Family can enhance or dampen, devastatingly, our interaction with this dimension of psyche. How, then, best creatively to anchor the individual in this sea of Otherness within which he or she swims psychospiritually?

The Object Relational Coniunctio

Thus attention to the depths of psyche draws us into the open outside world as much as it draws us down into the personal darkness of our personal experience. It pulls us toward other people and involvement in their lives as much as it withdraws us from them into pondering the images of a dream or the fantasies that arise from meditation.

—Ulanov 1986, 91

A relationship arrives de novo and lasts forever.

—Carl Whitaker,
in Neill and Kniskern 1982, 116

In my practice, I increasingly feel that analysis is incomplete until patients have grounded their work back into their families of origin and procreation (terms used by family theorists to describe one's birth family and one's marital or current relational family). I have found a useful weld between work done by what are now known as the intergenerational family therapists and Jungian analysts. It is interesting to me that, in the past several decades, both movements have been accelerating their approach to each other through the medium of a reassessed and enhanced object relations and self theory. Both schools exhibit a robust interest in the works of Kohut, Winnicott, Klein, Fairbairn, Sullivan, Mahler—all theorists who have noticed and reflected upon the profound impact of early family life-generated artifacts and imagoes in the formation of the ego-Self-Other synthesis (see esp., Framo 1992, 111–28; M. Stein 1982, 68–85).

No one questions the profound impact the object relations school has had upon the development of the analytical psychology movement. Many other traditional and innovative mental health movements have tapped into the same pragmatic reservoir of dynamic, structural, and interactive practice wisdom. The family therapy movement has been especially activated by object relational thinking in the past decade; their participation has effected substantial and elegant reformations of basic theory and approach. Across the object relational "bridge," Jungian analysts and family systems theorists can most readily meet and embrace each other (Slipp 1984).

Key to both systemic object relational and Jungian worldviews is a recent reinvigoration of transference conceptualizations and—most importantly—methodologies. However, the trick in relational uses of this very fertile depth phenomenon is the aiming and plotting of the therapeutic trajectory. In intense, individual work, that trajectory is always low-arched and immediate—enfolded in the projections and projective identifications of the analyst/analysand container. It is more concentrated, focused, and, in that way, somehow more relaxed and controlled. The cathartic intensity can build and implode/explode according to the cycles discovered in the analytic process.

Systemic transference, though rooted in the same individually mediated archetypal powers, possesses a higher arched, more diffuse, less contained trajectory. It is higher arched because it has the lift and propulsion of so many participants, all crowding onto the same therapeutic launch pad. Transferential explosives are ignited and potentially blown sky-high in such an intense environment.

In fact, the best wizards of systemic therapy (Haley, Minuchin, Whitaker, and Papp, for instance) look for ways to orchestrate and creatively trigger such propulsiveness (see esp., Gurman and Kniskern 1981, 1991; Nichols 1984). Whereas, in individual work, the therapist seeks to be the target and co-author of the projective and transference processes, in systemic work the therapist seeks more to appreciate, direct, and monitor the process. Therapists still participate; no one can avoid being projectively absorbed, as the alchemists have taught us, but it is not so personally arresting and consequential. The therapist notes and excites the transference realities; once these realities are noted and activated, the therapist returns them to the family system field, to blend them with the family's communal transferences. The therapist provokes and stands back, letting the system incubate its own transformative alternatives.

Unlike an analyst working with an individual, the family therapist may never have the pleasure of co-experiencing, in the same time-and space frame, the transformative fruits of this colabor with the family. Rather, the family therapist artfully seeds the system and sends it home, where the real, reabsorbed transference fruit is digested within the more relaxed and organic developmental cycles of ongoing family life.

Commingled and implicated with the transference mechanism is another core integrative concept—projective identification. However, it is a projective identification cast in the broader and bolder reconfigurations of recent years. Melanie Klein's original elaborations of nearly five decades ago have undergone impressive new theoretical adjustments. Among depth theorists, for example, Schwartz-Salant plays provocatively with this concept in his formulations on the "subtle-body couple" concept (1988). Among systemicists, the Scharff team emphasizes the "real-relational-world" dynamics of the concept (as opposed to its intrasubjective stress in the psychoanalytic literature) as it functions to bring both madness and meaning to relationship. Jill Scharff brilliantly and succinctly observes:

> I conclude that, in the family context, multiple individual processes governed by shared unconscious assumptions about family life eventually lead to the identification of parts of family experience inside individual personalities. At the same time, the intrapsychic situation is projected onto the intrafamilial group unconscious. An individual is selected as host for, or object for projection of, the disavowed parts of the central self of the family. In healthy families the host role rotates among the members, but when projective identification focuses and fixes on one member, a pathological situation has arisen, with an index person standing for a family group problem in metabolizing unwanted parts of the family group unconscious. (1992, 37–8)

Such a comprehensive merger of theoretical fields opens up a new universe of dialogue about the intrapsychic and interpersonal dimensions of the therapeutic process. In fact, analysis helps a person indexed as a static, "scapegoated" host to call upon personal and archetypal resources to permit a shift not just of intrapsychic position but of interpersonal position as well. Analysis propels individual and family complex rigidities and pathologies into new, more resilient and functional configurations. There is broadened analytic interest in the object relational way we literally get under each other's psychic skin through family inter-experience. Therapeutically, what results is what Framo describes as a "re-contouring of internal objects," and a reanimation of the phenomenally "real" outer family. The outer family frequently has become listless and defeated under the often decades-long, relentless droning of these ancient introjectively and projectively identified voices of despair and pain (Framo 1992, 117, 119).

Incest and Triangulation

> *A family is like a gun. If you point it in the wrong direction somebody is going to get killed.*
>
> *—Matthew Slaughter character in Hal Hartley's film,* Trust

> *It is not incestuous cohabitation that is desired but rebirth.*
>
> *—Jung, quoted in R. Stein 1973, 32*

Now that we have an archetypal model of family systems operation, and a developmental, object relations image of this process moving across the life cycle, how can we express the catalytic activator of this process? Again, the universal and unavoidable incest dynamic fills this activator role well. An interesting, almost provocative, operational parallel exists between Jung's notion of the complex and the intergenerationalist's insight into triangulation. For both theory structures, the crucial conceptual hinge is the dynamic of psychological incest. Increasingly, the perspective is that psychological incest and its developmental absorption and transformation will come to be seen as primary in our psychotherapeutic culture—more primary even than gender in the process of identity formation and individuation.

Triangulation is one of the most universally accepted theoretical concepts in the systemic therapies. It was "discovered," almost simultaneously, in a number of independent research and treatment facilities across the United States in the 1950s. But it was Murray Bowen who gave triangulation its most widely accepted orthodox description and application (Bowen 1978, 238–9, 273–6; Kerr and Bowen 1988, 134–62). The classical definition of triangulation is the way a weaker-resourced, third-person "scapegoat" is co-opted when a relational dyad develops a threatening instability. A common example is of a marital couple at a severe intimacy impasse, reaching across generations to one of their children and "triangling" that child as a deflector and dissipator of marital despair.

For example, mother teaches high school during the day and is a city councilwoman at night. Father is left at home evenings, alone with the responsibility of child care and home maintenance. He feels increasingly lonely and resentful. He attempts to entice mother sexually when she comes home late; she says she is too tired for sexual play. He flies into a rage and threatens divorce. Mother flees their bedroom and sleeps with her two oldest daughters. Next week their oldest daughter, thirteen years old, is found intoxicated with two boys in an alley in a high crime district of town. The parents pick up their daughter up at the juvenile receiving center, take her home, and then berate her shameful behavior. The parents have successfully, and unconsciously, triangulated and deflected/projected their relational impasse upon their scapegoated daughter.

This inter-generational "perverse triangle" (Gurman and Kniskern 1981, 279) is a very compelling construct—inherently unstable, fluid, and, most essentially, unavoidable. After his early years of recognition of and fascination with family triangulation patterns, Bowen went to Jane Goodall's African research station to watch primates in their natural jungle habitat:

> I just sat up in those trees watching those monkeys through binoculars with Jane and was amazed to discover that monkeys triangulate just like humans—the whole damn mammal world triangulates it would seem. Amazing. (Bowen 1981)

Bowen's view of this ontogenetic, mammalian triangle is profound. The triangle is a major adaptational safety valve—"where anxiety increases, a third person becomes involved in the tension of the twosome, creating a triangle . . . . [The triangle] decreases anxiety by spreading it through the system." This new "interconnected" triangulate whole has a much greater capacity to hold anxiety than the sum of the former separate family unit members, "because pathways are in place that allow the shifting of anxiety around the system." Therefore, the triangle is more stable than the often more volatile dyad in the essential "anxiety-binding process" that lies at the core of human inter-personal survival (Kerr and Bowen 1988, 135).

In function, triangles are eternal. Though their content is constantly shifting, their form is dynamically and often perniciously enduring. They outlive their creators. Grandchildren act out the remnant reactive processes of their dead grandparents. Triangles are the "building blocks" of family "chaos." In the face of the most traumatic of family stress events, this "anxiety-induced loss of differentiation" becomes so taxing that not only do single-unit triangulations occur, but complex interlocking systemic triangulations are brought into play (Kerr and Bowen 1988, 134–42).

Bowen discovered systemic triangulations unexpectedly, during clinical observations behind a psychoanalytic mental hospital's one-way mirror. Courageously, he explored this powerful experimental concept and applied it to his own family of origin. Resistance to his personal family amplifications ran so high that he had to present his original professional paper on this topic to his colleagues under disguised conditions. Later, they were published in "anonymous" form (Framo 1972, 111–73). In this pioneering effort, Bowen discovered that what transforms the pernicious drain of multi-generational triangulations is the building of a conscious awareness of and presence to the triangulating matrix of family itself. This crucial process he called differentiation. He created a "coaching" process wherein persons were carefully educated in methods to re-enter, non-reactively and dyadically, the "undifferentiated family ego mass" (Framo 1972, 113) of their originating families without surrendering their conscious calm, perspective, and sense of well-being. Bowen's model, as further elaborated by Framo, Friedman, and Williamson, serves as the major basis for my analytical elaborations of this powerful technique (Framo 1992; Friedman 1985; Williamson 1991).

This triangulation process is one half of the central psyche-systems synthesis which I advocate. The omnipresent incest dynamic is the other. The incest theme was indisputably a driving theoretical and methodological vision for Jung, especially in the years of his mature clinical formulation, from 1912 onward. Incest was the burning match that incinerated his close bond with Freud, in the 1911 and 1912 publications of what eventually became *Symbols of Transformation* (Jung 1967). Incest-libido work was still central to his thinking in his late career—so central that he extensively revised *Symbols of Transformation* in 1951.

From the beginning, Jung was aware of his deep psychic fascination with incest issues. He warned Freud in the fall of 1910 to "be prepared for something strange the likes of which has never yet been heard from me" (Wehr 1987, 133). Looking back at that portentous publishing event from the vantage point of his 1951 revision, Jung commented, "I was acutely conscious, then, of the loss of friendly relations with Freud and of the lost comradeship of our work together" (Jung 1967, *xxvi*). All of this was brewing in the same vat of *prima materia* experience as Jung's now well-documented affairs with Sabina Spielrein and Toni Wolff. Incest dynamics course through every thread of the complex weave of these relationships: the homoerotic bond (of that nascent, inspiring variety found between creatively engaged fathers and sons) between Jung and Freud; Jung's cranky defensiveness over the ethical breach with Spielrein ("She [Spielrein] has caused a nasty scandal for me, simply because I chose to forgo the pleasure of begetting a child with her"); and the intense, post-Freud break involvement with Toni Wolff, in which Wolff arguably functioned both as lover-therapist and as mediator of the central Jungian anima construct (Weir 1985, 138–43 and 187–90; Carotenuto 1980).

The intergenerationalist would see in these charged events the strong possibility of a determined, though proto-conscious, effort on Jung's part to shatter the remnant incestuous attachments of his family of origin—where the pre-Oedipal Jung lived in a home atmosphere permeated by the broodings of seriously symptomatic parents—and subsequent projective parental figures, most notably Freud (see esp., Weir 1987, 31–8, 47–54, 138–45). The relationship-shattering quality of these publications and affairs served to distance the devouring threat of key incest figures in much the same way that people are emotionally "cut off," often violently and finally, from this same regressive incest pressure within their families of origin (Kerr and Bowen 1988, 271–81). Jung eventually came consciously to understand the deep, psychoid power of these mechanisms, and theorized brilliantly about them. He came to understand that these were complexes—charged, feeling-toned, psychic asteroids of great numinous power. And he realized that they floated around freely in the matrix of repressed personal experience and the collective inheritances of the Objective Psyche. He knew that individuation would come only with their conscious confrontation and transformation.

By 1912, Jung understood these complexes as issuing originally from the incestuous womb of the Great Mother, the organic engine of regression, absorption, and ultimate personal annihilation—unless one consciously sojourns back within the Great Mother to find the slumbering Divine Child "awaiting his [sic] conscious realization":

> [T]herapy must support the regression, and continue to do so until the "prenatal" stage is reached. It must be remembered that the "mother" is really an imago, a psychic image merely. . . . The "mother" as the first incarnation of the anima archetype, personifies in fact the whole unconscious. Hence the regression leads back only apparently to the mother; in reality she is the gateway into the unconscious, into the "realm of the Mothers." (Jung 1967, par. 508)

The incest complex, if left unanalyzed and unconfronted, keeps us chained forever to the regressive instincts; it paradoxically creates the very kind of death that incestuous clinging seeks to avoid: "The neurotic who cannot leave his mother has good reason to do so: ultimately it is the fear of death that holds him there" (Jung 1967, par. 415). The essential therapeutic aspect of each individual's psychic growth is consciously to face this regressive, incestuous substrate in all of our experience, and to mature through, suffer through, and evolve through the struggle of that encounter. All of us need to be "dissolved in 'friendly water'. . . which is equated with the maternal womb and corresponds to the *prima materia*" (Edinger 1985, 48). Incest is the key transforming alchemical operation of individuation. This individuation process has both a literal, real-family-world dynamic and an archetypal, mythic-family-world dynamic. Any therapy which attends only to one portion of this equation is partial and incomplete.

As always with Jung, the solution to this massive incest lure is a conscious return to the archetypal, incestuous world of the unconscious. Without such an individuating journey, one cannot gain the "non-specific" instinctual nectar of libido and its sexual, self-preservative, spiritual, and aesthetic flowerings in the psyche (Jacoby 1990, 34). But as visceral and earthy as this language and these metaphors seem to be, they apparently worked for Jung at the symbolic level only. The possibility of a literal return and transformative connection to the actual, biological family of origin, and introjectively enfleshed mothers and fathers, is often subtly disparaged:

> The development of consciousness inevitably leads not only to separation from the mother, but to separation from the parents and the whole family circle and thus to a relative degree of detachment from the unconscious and the world of instinct. (Jung 1967, par. 351)

Jung discovered that incest is an imaginal opportunity as much as a symptomatic affliction. Like many of the current transgenerational family therapists, he came to appreciate that the incest dynamic is embedded in the developmental process. It is a key activator of major phases in psychic maturation. It becomes an abortive dynamic when it becomes literalized and reductive. The incestuous, transgenerational chemistry is an imaginal chemistry, a medium-of-image through which parental love embeds in the child the deepest soul contents of both personal and archetypal learnings.

It is not surprising that a materialist culture like ours has literalized and deformed this symbolic matrix. Incest is seen only as an illegal evil, to be hunted down and eradicated by the well-meaning but often soulless bureaucratic legions of child protective services. The old Hermetic wisdoms of ages past are discarded in such a positivist world view. The universal, symbolic incest process is a mystical process, a child of the ancient *anima mundi*—the non-dualist, holistic world where both spirit and matter couple, create, and reproduce ever more healing image-processes. Without question, we must stop the devastating enactments of *literal* childhood sexual and physical abuse, with their withering, enduring torments to the child's, and future adult's soul. But, just as urgently, we must differentially seek never to cripple or interfere with the imaginal, alchemical, developmental, and spiritually benevolent aspects of the psychological incest process. Wise, vibrant cultures know the difference. Brutal, immature cultures blur the difference.

The intergenerational family therapists confirm, from an independent line of insight and therapeutic technique, the same crucial importance of the incest dynamic. They would readily agree with Jung that "a new adaptation or orientation of vital importance can only be achieved in accordance with the instincts" (Jung 1967, par. 351). But they would disagree that this transformative event can occur only with archetypal compensation beyond the actual unconscious bonds and attachments of the originating biological family matrix. For them, the instinctual can work its transformative magic only through a literal return to that family medium, from within the chrysalis of a new stance or attitude. Literal return is unavoidable if transformative change, the Jungian individuation or the Bowenian differentiation, is to occur.

Triangulation. The incest complex. The fuel is the same: incestuous family bonding. For Jung, the complex casts its spell across that mysterious hinterland between the personal and the archetypal unconscious—a conduit and bridge, at one and the same moment allowing for the personal and the mythic, the individual and the collective, to meet and reify, to ignite the fire of consciousness or to annihilate the unaware soul.

For the inter-generationalist, the triangle is equally portentous. Bowen felt it to be a universal experience across all of the known mammal species, and maybe the entire biosphere (Bowen 1981). It is the frontier between generations. It is that liminal zone where the species-future and the ancestral past encounter and provoke each other. It is the touchstone of species-memory and anticipation, the housing of the family's psychic DNA, the place where the next generation is bound and coerced, instructed and prepared. Triangulation is unavoidable. It is the central organ of generational transmission and enablement. Triangulation can crush one's individuated destiny and differentiation, or can fulfill it.

Individuation/differentiation, seen from this broader perspective, depends on the right balance of systemic forces and an individual attitude of nonreactive calm. Only within the embrace of such a synthesis can an individual consciously flow through the familial labyrinth, across both individual and family life cycles. We cannot individuate just intrapsychically but must, with equal conviction and intensity, "reciprocate fully, both backward and forward through time" with our families, if we are "to experience well being" (Williamson and Bray 1988, 366). The flesh of the Objective Psyche derives its very life and continuity from both of these sources. In fact, the inner complex almost inevitably "fires" in reaction to outer triangulations. These two processes are opposite faces of the same processual coin. For both Bowen and Jung, there is profound appreciation for the dynamic and often volatile flow of unceasing complex activity in both the individual and family psyche. To remain unconscious and passive in this living stream of ancestral being is to remain a vulnerable victim of blind individual and family fate.

A Synthesis Model: Systemization Mirroring Individuation

> *People change. Not everything stays with you all of your life.*
>
> *—Emilina Domingos, in Barbara Kingsolver's* Animal Dreams, *1988*

Psyche unfolds both within our skins and without. Psyche produces consciousness within our personal experience and beyond. Individuals—and the families of which they are an inextricable part—mature, evolve, go crazy, regress, and transform. There is individuation and differentiation, within a depth system both intrapsychic and interpersonal at once. The depth task cannot avoid the responsibility of seeking, theoretically and operationally, to blend these two process-twins.

My cross-generational work, within a clearly defined analytical context, seeks to respect both the inner-familial, mythic aspects of the incest dynamic and the outer-familial, systemic aspects of the triangulating dynamism outlined above. The actual "live" cross-generational encounters are usually positioned near the end of the analytical experience, because I am profoundly aware of the immense family-systemic and mythic-archetypal energies which are aroused by such a direct and unveiled exploration of these ancient affects. Lighting such a psychic firestorm intentionally needs careful therapeutic preparation and protection. Both Freud and Jung recognized the essential role of the incest dynamic in shaping and motivating the psyche and its destiny. To approach this dynamic without careful analytic awareness and sensitivity would be dangerous and potentially devastating folly. The intergenerational theorists have shown us that to approach this same incestuous vortex without a careful systemic awareness could provoke an equally devastating result.

The intergenerational model is a genuinely systemic/relational model and is temperamentally best suited for the analytic frame. Bowen's coaching model of working with families "at a distance" is the foundational approach (Framo 1972, 127–8). Acutely aware of the disruptive power of reactive anxieties and triangulations within the family-of-origin matrix, Bowen found that a period of careful, almost didactic, preparation of patients for encounters with their families is crucial. Using his now famous innovation of the family genogram (a schematic family tree), Bowen clearly traces multi-generational patterns of triangulations and reactive anxieties—going back at least three generations—which have ensnared the family field (McGoldrick and Gerons, 1985). He behaviorally rehearses both the information and its impact for the patient in these sessions. He uses the genogram to instruct and to relieve cognitively (by discharging unconsciously generated anxieties often decades old). It is overtly a cognitive model, through which Bowen attempts to get the patient to think about family dynamics as a way to avoid affective possession and inducement to unconscious repetitions. I find the genogram invaluable not only in mapping out the obvious patterns of triangulation but also in expressing the mythic and complex fields which also "possess" the family. When patients were ready, Bowen sent them home to their families of origin. These visits were carefully prepared for, and the agendas were kept painstakingly circumscribed and focused (Richardson 1984; Kerr and Bowen 1988; Gurman and Kniskern 1981; Kerr 1993).

Donald Williamson, in an often sharp revision of Bowen's process, has framed this coaching movement in therapy as a preparatory phase to live family "consultations" (Williamson 1981, 1982a, 1982b, 1991). As patients gain insight (in therapeutic small groups) into the family force field, they are instructed to write practice letters and make practice audio tapes, in preparation for sending actual letters and tapes. This whole process culminates in the invitation to parents to participate in an intensive, multi-day, intergenerational consultation.

Though the authors of this consultative mode of intergenerational family work vary as to the form and content of preparatory and live family sessions, certain factors are consistent across methodologies. All emphasize the care needed to conduct these events. They are acutely aware of what analysis would describe as the complex-field in place when this transgenerational family comes together. All the power of the ancestors, of family archetypal pattern, and of unconscious family trauma pulsates in the consulting room during these visits. Everyone is terrified of blame and judgment being laid at their feet and, most of all, is terrified of the fear of irreparable disaster, which may result from attempting such a meeting in the first place. There is great apprehension that the truthful and personal telling of pain will annihilate rather than inform and heal. The therapist must proceed with great directive caution, humor, sensitivity, and genuine caring in order to dispel these ominous affective fears.

Most of these consultative modelers claim success (a) when the patient is able to navigate the experience not only in-tact but having exercised the non-reactive leadership they were tutored to accomplish and (b) when inappropriate generational boundary violations have been sealed and terminated. Williamson believes that this last factor focuses sharply on the culminating event: the adult patient child turning to his or her opposite-sexed parent in the physical presence of the same-sex parent, and clearly declaring that their love-affair is now terminated, and that she or he is autonomous of caretaking responsibility for this perseverating and debilitating transgenerational incest (Williamson 1981, 1982a, 1982b).

Analytic Improvisations on an Intergenerational Theme

> *I was in a vast train station, like Grand Central. I was scurrying all around in a frenzy . . . trying to find my son. I looked on platform after platform and he was not to be found. Then I saw him. He waved at me and touched me through the barricade and then he said, gently but firmly, that he had to go. I knew he was gone for good. And that it was okay somehow. I awoke in deep tears.*
>
> *—Dream of a mother during a family consultation process with her analytic patient son*

I have executed an analytic adaptation of these transgenerational models. Like Williamson and Framo especially, I use a flexible, eclectic approach within the solid, grounding structure of the analytic frame. This normally means that I build gradually toward the introduction of one-at-a-time family consultations with parents (and maybe siblings). However, I have changed these rules in special circumstances and seen people in all assemblages, from the full family to differing sub-system combinations. Or, I have simply coached patients in preparation for their own visits home to their families. What is presented here is a normative, not dogmatic, model.

Throughout these proceedings, the analyst functions primarily as facilitator, and guarantor that the family "consultants" are not violated or tricked into unfair revelations, vulnerabilities, and judgments. The patient is left primarily responsible for the content and accomplishment of the learning agenda, as rehearsed for many months or years in anticipation of this crucial sequence of dialogues. Scheduling sessions is critical, and should allow enough time between these hyper-intense encounters for family members to process both consciously and unconsciously, and to accommodate themselves to the inevitable and often massive shifts in individual and family self-images. All are told that the effects of the consultative event can be experienced in strong "flashbacks" of feeling and arousing images for a long time after the consultations. This process of normalization, and naming of the momentous nature of what they are undergoing, is followed by the warmly communicated readiness of the analyst to be available for subsequent continuing and "refresher" consultations if these are desired.

Admittedly, once the intergenerational encounter occurs, enormous therapeutic expectation is placed on the potential results of this interaction. The actual real-time, face-to-face experience is built on the careful, prefatory, analytical working of the unconscious materials, and on exploratory expressions of these new visions through "coached" letters, audio or video tapes, brief home visits, and family travels together (to places of historical, affective significance for the family, such as graves of ancestors, childhood homesites, etc.). Despite this preparation, the "live" encounter is always charged. For the invited family consultant it is inevitably a frightening experience to enter another family member's therapeutic space.

Normally, I structure at least two extended patient/ family member sessions with each parent and, often, with each sibling. As mentioned already, these intergenerational sessions are encouraged to occur near the end of mid- to long-term personal analysis, but the unpredictable turns and torque of the dynamic analytic process can warrant such sessions at about any stage of the process. For example, one analysand's mother contracted a rapidly progressing terminal cancer, and we necessarily and fruitfully conducted these sessions at the commencement of analysis. What is crucial above all else is that these sessions be carefully rehearsed and prepared for; if the patient is still significantly reactive and unconscious to much of the family complex-field, there is significant potential during these consultations for therapeutic harm and re-wounding of both the patient and family member(s). Responsible analytic use of these powerful systemic tools demands respect for the potentially devastating downside of the consultative encounter. A poorly contained "mega" therapeutic event like this can almost guarantee years of continued individual and family entropy, suffering, and avoidance—"We tried family therapy once and we were really hurt—it was awful."

In the ideal circumstance, the patient will bring in the family member consultant for a late Friday afternoon session of ninety minutes. Then, they are encouraged to play and enjoy themselves over the weekend, and to avoid much overt processing of the often volatile content introduced during the opening session. However, they are instructed to remember dreams and to privately record internal feelings, ideas, images, and questions that surface during the weekend. A follow-up session is held Monday morning, with both patient and family consultant, to process their reactions to the first encounter.

As analyst, I define myself as a facilitator during these sessions. The patient is clearly the convenor and director of the event. The patient describes, as rehearsed, why she or he came into therapy, and presides over the asking of the consultative questions. The visiting family member is genuinely thanked for his or her courage and generosity in attending such an unusual therapeutic gathering, and is given permission to say volumes or nothing at all in response to the questions asked, questions of real developmental moment and urgency raised by the patient. The family member is simply guaranteed that his or her role is purely consultative; he or she will not be tricked into any personal therapy or exposure. As analyst, I simply hold the frame, shape and deepen the process as helpfully as I can, and seek to prevent violation of the promised protective covenant and rules of engagement.

Most often, four question-clusters are explored in some depth during these family-of-origin consultations:

1. VOCATIONAL/DEVELOPMENTAL: How did the consultant handle such a crisis as the patient has been facing?

   "Dad, mom, I came into therapy feeling forlorn after my divorce at 38 and my job loss at 41. I felt suicidal and crazy—full of despair. Did you ever have such a crisis? If so, how did you handle it—how did you survive?"

2. RELATIONAL/SEXUAL: How did the consultant handle the relational life dilemmas the patient is struggling with?

   "Dad, Mom, I had three affairs during my marriage. The last one broke up my marriage. Did you ever have an affair or think about having one? If so, how did you process the deep strains and wild emotional surges of such an event in your life?"

3. INCESTUOUS: How did the consultant manage the strong incestuous pulls of the family-of-origin, pulls which the patient has discovered have survived into his or her adulthood and adult relationships?

   "Dad, I realize, as your oldest daughter, that I have strong, uncontested loyalties to you and deep fears of your disapproval if I violate those loyalties. I realize in many ways I am more 'wedded' and loyal to you than to my husband. I intend gracefully but firmly to end the unhelpful aspects of that loyalty this weekend. How did you deal with your incestuous loyalties to your mother?"

4. EXISTENTIAL: What does the consultant feel is the central purpose and destiny of her or his life?

   "Mom, Dad, what has been most important for you to accomplish in this life. Have you succeeded or failed? Are you ready for or afraid of your death? When do you imagine you will die and what shape will your life be in then?"

The patient is not ready for the consultation if she or he is not really intrigued by, interested in, and open to the depth answer of the consultant. Families fear these areas of inquiry. They have rarely openly alluded to these contents and depths. They have instinctually known that such questions open the doors to the family unconscious—to the secrets and terrors that have lain there, unseen and unprocessed, often for generations. The questions terrify and mesmerize. The patient is instructed to keep these questions open-ended and non-accusatory. They must be asked carefully, in a therapeutic temenos that is contemplative, respectful, patient, and gentle, for they open up the very psychic bedrock of the reproductive and purposive urges of the species.

The case study that follows is a cameo of a courageously disclosed inner-family domain of soul. It is an example of implementing the coaching model described earlier. Unlike much of my analytic work, where the intergenerational encounters are staged live in my office, the real life encounters for this patient occurred in visits to her European home. Hers is a useful illustration of the rich and manifold adaptations possible using the basic systemic, intergenerational principles within analytic practice. It also features a way that analysts practicing in traditional formats could begin to integrate and adapt the analytic container to absorb some useful and powerful systemic notions about the life of the family psyche. I am deeply grateful to this patient for her willingness to share her intergenerational ancestral journey. Of course, the case study is masked to maintain confidentiality.

The Secret

Gretchen arrived in my lobby pert, coiffed, and controlled. Her impeccable diction was deepened by the residual charm of her native German tongue, lightly and melodiously accenting the stream of her English speech. She was cosmopolitan. She was Vogue. She was Dietrich, pre-war Berlin.

Gretchen was also deeply dysphoric, and adrift inside that

cosmopolitan mosaic. After deploying an initial flare of precise and coy reasons for having had sought out analysis with me, she grew wary, tight, and pensive. Long silences filled our encounter. Very early on, her eyes became haunted, almost vacant. She stared guardedly at me as though at a specter from out of the past: "Your eyes . . . they are like my husband's eyes . . . so wounded . . . it scares me to look at them . . . I cry . . . I hate to cry," she told me in simple agony.

She remembered a dream of entering her bedroom and finding, there in the corner, an old, cheap curtain which she pulled apart. There she discovered another room with a bare, harshly-glaring light bulb dangling by a frayed cord from an unfinished attic ceiling. Below it sat her husband in a dirty T-shirt and underwear. He was unshaven and somnolent, sitting in an unkempt, despairing silence:

> He was horrible looking. His eyes were bulging out and he was emaciated. He was starring at me but he almost looked dead. He resembled one of those guys from Buchenwald . . . . I screamed . . . . I could not remove my eyes from his horrible looking eyes and face. I thought, "What have I done to him.?"

This was the "real" Gretchen, undoubtedly carried and projectively identified with by her repressed husband. This was the unkempt, somnolent aspect of her deeply wounded inner self that she had kept hidden in the closet behind the culture and poise of her outer-world persona. This was the shell-shocked remnant of infantile intrusions upon the sanctity of the Self. Beneath Gretchen's outer vivacity and charm sat this impoverished, famished, lost, narcissistic soul.

She amplified this material to memories of her father's distant despair. He held some still unrevealed secret about an earlier marriage "which we all discovered after I had been in the family for quite some time. A government census office had called and said my mother's and his marriage was invalid because he had not gotten a legal divorce from his first wife. I was illegitimate overnight. And we had known nothing of all of this! So much of him is secret, hidden. His emptiness feels like mine. If he won't talk, somehow I cannot really speak either."

And, so, the problem of Gretchen's living, the problem in her psyche, was both an inner impoverishment and a mirroring outer familial impoverishment. An empty, outer father/husband fed and contributed to an inner emaciation and despair. To treat one necessarily required treating the other. Therapy is Janus-headed, looking both outward and inward all of the time, sometimes sequentially but sometimes—maddeningly—simultaneously. This poignant image of her outer paternal pain and her inner masculine vacancy claimed a dual regard in my treatment plans and images for our work together. Effective analysis had to treat both the inner father-complex and the outer real-father relationship. The psyche was frozen by both the paralyzing introject and the mesmerizing project.

Early in the therapeutic process, I began gently coaching Gretchen in ways to interact not only with the wisdom of her inner psyche but with the outer-relational, familial psyche as well. She was to cast a disciplined and caring eye on both her dream life and her family-of-origin life. She wrote down her dreams and she wrote to her parents. The early work was delicate. Gretchen was testy, touchy about the slightest actual or perceived empathic violations. She wavered about her commitment to analysis, threatening at almost every session to end "this silly mistake. This is too painful, it just isn't the right time for me."

But, then, over a year into the process, the psyche began to manifest itself vibrantly after a long series of desolation dreams (such as the one about her staring, starving husband). She dreamed of entering "a huge Gothic cathedral . . . so high and large that it was breathtaking." She was dancing and talking with a Jewish woman "about the suffering that she, as a Jew, had experienced, the rejections, the pain"; but, "also the bonding of her people and the joy she experienced in the dances and the music." She was in Buddhist temples full of light and mystery. She was in ancient Goddess circles and ceremonies around fire and blood and sacrament. The Self was alive indeed after years of abuse and repression. The deep soul had survived intact and the ego knew where the connecting paths still could be found.

Gretchen experienced childhood in a cramped suburban Berlin apartment. This apartment brooded with a daily office of compulsive risings and retirings, inane work, and stifling affective silences. The blood of the family emotional organism grew more and more anemic over the years—especially after the secret of the father's past family intruded into the present family's conscious psychic sphere. Parental repression and affective disavowals were harsh and sometimes punitive. For the first time in her life, Gretchen was letting something else into those eviscerating family quarters, as exemplified by this poignant dream vignette:

> *At that point it was as if there were no longer two cars, but Terry [the analyst] and I were sitting one behind the other in the car. I could feel his body against mine. I could feel his penis against my leg. I could feel it become alive and grow against me. We sat there for awhile. I thought I could not take the closeness. I did not want it for fear . . . . I came out of the car and went home, that is, in my parents [old, childhood] apartment. It was summertime. The windows in the dining room were wide open. I looked through the window to see if Terry would leave. He did not. I stayed in the dining room wondering what to do. In a way I wanted him to leave because of my fears; on the other hand I was hoping he would stay. My parents' place seemed to be a very secure place. I heard a car leave. I looked out the window to see if it was Terry. It was another car. I saw Terry still sitting in his car. I still had strong mixed feelings. I wanted him to go, yet I wanted him to stay and I so wanted to be able to run downstairs to go and be with him.*

A new season had fallen across the inner and outer familial apartment. New windows of eros and relation were open. New penises of insight, passion, and promise were penetrating secret complexes and tyrannies. Ego was still frozen in fear, but now ego was at least imagining running after new loves and destinies.

All the while, Gretchen was writing to her family and taking extended visits to her childhood home in Germany. She was imagining in analysis the "feeling-questions" and fearful things she would like to explore with her sister, mother, and father during these visits. Paradoxically, she alternatively felt much more anxious on these home visits and, "sometimes as calm as I've ever been, there or anywhere," as she non-reactively asked provocative consultative questions, especially of her parents. As Gretchen gained insight and mastery in dialogue with her complex-self, she gained mastery of her environmental self as well. The two were simultaneously building and reinforcing energies.

Eventually, Gretchen decided to explode the family secret: "I know I have half-siblings somewhere. I am going to find them and tell them what I know of the past and ask them for what they know. My parents' terror can no longer control my life." This flowering self-assertion followed a dramatic dream of finding a lost child in a dungeon (the French word in her dream was *oubliettes*) or catacomb, in the side of a hill. Gretchen found this child and awoke as she was trying to lure the weary waif into the light: "The lock was broken, the child was free to go but still she was terrified to leave that awful place. I feel so much connection with and sorrow for her—so much grief." Gretchen was becoming her own child protective services worker. Interestingly, the French derivation of the word *oubliettes* is medieval. It was the underground dungeon in castles where the political and debtor prisoners were kept. The word literally means "forgotten." Gretchen was recovering the forgotten parts of her soul and lost innocence which had been languishing in an unconscious inter-projective prison.

Creatively utilizing our analytic coaching process and entrepreneurially tracking therapeutic resources in Germany, Gretchen choreographed a dramatic event. She gathered the family and defined the structure and agenda. Firmly and without inflaming her parents, she asked to learn all that her father and mother knew of the past and of the lost family of half-siblings. She asserted her right to connection with these forgotten blood kin.

Gretchen discovered that her mother, out of the raw fear of change, was even more invested in maintaining the secret, and the isolation than was her father. Over the next year, Gretchen, and her now fully mobilized sister, rifled government records for leads. Eventually, she located the half-siblings and choreographed poignant reunions. Throughout, she met regularly with both her parents and sister (in whole family sessions and one-on-one encounters). Rather than provoking the heart-attack or death of one or both of her aging parents that Gretchen had feared, she instead discovered that, for her father at least, a new vibrancy of inner life and interpersonal resilience emerged. Only her mother grew more neurotic and brooding—another clear indication of the mother's masked but prominent collaborative role in architecting the years of childhood emotional abuse and restraint. The unhealthy, incestuous collaborations of this family system were opened up to new developmental horizons by Gretchen's conscious, non-reactive labors.

Familius imaginalis

The family is the place where there are life and death voltages.
—Carl Whitaker, in Framo 1992, 60

Literature as a panacea for couples in distress.
—Oudalle, in Michel Tournier's "The Taciturn Lovers," 1991

Family work in analysis never has to be literal. It often is most powerful as an imaginal presence. James Hillman is correct in his repeated clarion call for a reanimation of the world, a real re-ensouling of our shared phenomenal existence. The Renaissance rediscovered this *anima mundi* and so must we (Hillman 1983, 1985). The lens of the imagination is the lens of the Divine, bringing our senses back to consciousness of the dance of the gods, which permeates all aspects of our existence.

Family systems theory is a crucial new thread to add to the weave of our intrapsychic work. In outer-world motion and emotion it mirrors, enhances, and completes inner-world motion and emotion. Like the twin snakes of the staff of Asclepius, family systems theory and Jungian analytical theory complement each other, embroidering the trunk of a fully lived psyche. The ancestors live not only in the images of the objective unconscious, as mediated by our complexes and dreams, but also in the behaviors and interactions of our current family realities. A holistic therapy looks in both places. It works in both places. It connects both movements of human endeavor and soul.

Psyche lives everywhere. Psyche's alchemy is a true chemistry for all living processes, individual and collective. If the Jungian hermeneutic is coherent, pliant, and elegantly simple enough to have a wide-ranging application across the vast divides of the intricate universe, it must be extended into all realms of experience, intrapsychically and interpsychically. And, the place where Psyche lives perhaps most abundantly is in the family and in its vast restorative powers of curative, collective imaginings.

References

Bertine, Eleanor 1992. *Close Relationships: Family, Friendship, Marriage.* Toronto: Inner City Books.

Boszormenyi-Nagy, I., and Krasner, B. 1986. *Between Give and Take.* New York: Brunner/Mazel.

Bowen, M. 1978. *Family Therapy in Clinical Practice.* New York: Jason Aronson.

———. 1981. Seminar: Intergenerational Family Therapy. Sponsored by Seattle Family Institute, Seattle, WA. December 4–5, 1981.

Campbell, J. 1988. *Historical Atlas of World Mythology.* Vols. 1 and 2. New York: Harper and Row.

Carotenuto, A. 1982. *A Secret Symmetry: Sabina Spielrein between Freud and Jung.* London: Routledge and Kegan Paul.

Dodson, L. 1983. Intertwining Jungian depth psychology and family therapy through use of action techniques. *Journal of Group Psychotherapy, Psychodrama and Sociometry.* Winter Issue: 155–64.

Edinger, E. 1985. *Anatomy of the Psyche: Alchemical Symbolism in Psychotherapy.* LaSalle, Ill.: Open Court Press.

Ekstrom, S. 1988. The family as context for the individuation process: A Jungian approach for working with the family. *The Family; Personal, Cultural and Archetypal Dimensions: Proceedings from the National Conference of Jungian Analysts, 1988.* San Francisco: C. G. Jung Institute of San Francisco. 79–93.

Eliade, M. 1978. *A History of Religious Ideas.* Vols. 1–3. Chicago: University of Chicago Press.

Framo, J. L. 1972. *Family Interaction: A Dialogue Between Family Research and Family Therapy.* New York: Springer Publications.

———. 1992. *Family-of-Origin Therapy: An Intergenerational Approach.* New York: Brunner/Mazel.

Friedman, E. 1985. *Generation to Generation: Family Process in Church and Synagogue.* New York: Guilford Press.

Guggenbühl-Craig, A. 1986. *Marriage: Dead or Alive.* Dallas: Spring.

Gurman, A. S., and Kniskern, D. P. 1981. *Handbook of Family Therapy.* New York: Brunner/Mazel.

———. 1991. *Handbook of Family Therapy.* Vol. 2. New York: Brunner/Mazel.

Hall, J. A. and Young-Eisendrath, P. 1988. *The Book of the Self.* New York: New York University Press.

Hillman, J. 1983. *Archetypal Psychology: A Brief Account.* Dallas: Spring.

———. 1985. *Anima: An Anatomy of a Personified Notion.* Dallas: Spring.

———. 1992. *We've Had a Hundred Years of Psychotherapy and the World's Getting Worse.* San Francisco: Harper.

Jacoby, M. 1990. *Individuation and Narcissism: The Psychology of the Self in Jung and Kohut.* London: Routledge.

Jung, C. G. 1973. Answer to Job. In *CW* 11. Princeton: Princeton University Press.

———. 1970. *Mysterium Coniunctionis. CW* 14. Princeton: Princeton University Press.

———. 1968. *Aion. CW* 9.ii. Princeton: Princeton University Press.

———. 1967. *Symbols of Transformation. CW* 5. Princeton: Princeton University Press.

———. 1963. *Memories, Dreams and Reflections.* New York: Pantheon.

Kerr, M. 1993. Seminar: Addictions and the family. Sponsored by the Center for the Family, Santa Rosa, CA. June 25 and 26, 1993.

Kerr, M. E., and Bowen M. 1988. *Family Evaluation: The Role of the Family as an Emotional Unit that Governs Individual Behavior and Development.* New York: W. W. Norton & Co.

Lacan, J. 1977. *Ecrits: A Selection.* Trans. A. Sheridan. New York: W. W. Norton.

Masson, J. M. 1986. Freud and the child sexual abuse controversy. Paper presented at the Freud and and the Origins of Psychoanalysis Lecture-Discussion Series, University of Washington Extension, Seattle, WA. November 25, 1986.

McGoldrick, M., and Gerons, R. 1985. *Genograms in Family Assessment.* New York: W. W. Norton & Co.

Neil, J. R., and Kniskern, D. P., eds. 1982. *From Psyche to System: The Evolving Therapy of Carl Whitaker.* New York: Guilford Press.

Nichols, M. 1984. *Family Therapy: Concept and Methods.* New York: Gardner Press.

Papadopoulos, R., and Saayman, G. 1990. Towards a Jungian approach to family therapy. *Harvest: Journal for Jungian Studies* 35 (1989–90): 95–120.

Rutter, P. 1989. *Sex in the Forbidden Zone.* Los Angeles: Jeremy P. Tarcher.

Richardson, Ronald W. 1984. *Family Ties That Bind.* Vancouver, B.C.: Self Counsel Series.

Samuels, A. 1985. *Jung and the Post-Jungians.* London: Routledge and Kegan Paul.

Scharff, D. E., and Scharff, J. S. 1991. *Object Relations Couple Therapy*. Northvale, N. J.: Jason Aronson.

Scharff, J. S. 1992. *Projective and Introjective Identification and the Use of the Therapist's Self*. Northvale, N. J.: Jason Aronson.

Schwartz-Salant, N. 1988. *The Borderline Personality: Vision and Healing*. Wilmette, Ill.: Chiron Publications.

Slipp, S. 1984. *Object Relations: A Dynamic Bridge Between Individual and Family Treatment*. New York.: Jason Aronson.

Stein, M., ed. 1982. *Jungian Analysis*. La Salle, Ill.: Open Court.

Stone, H. and Winkelman, S. 1989. *Embracing Each Other: Relationship as Teacher, Healer and Guide*. San Rafael, Calif.: New World Library.

Stein, R. 1973. *Incest and Human Love*. New York: The Third Press.

Tournier, M. 1991. *The Midnight Love Feast*. London: Collins.

Ulanov, A. B. 1986. *Picturing God*. Cambridge, Mass.: Cowley Publications.

Wehr, G. 1987. *Jung: A Biography*. Boston: Shambhala.

Williamson, D. S. 1991. *The Intimacy Paradox: Personal Authority in the Family System*. New York: Guilford Press.

———. 1981. Personal authority via termination of the intergenerational hierarchical boundary: A new stage in the family life cycle. *Journal of Marriage and Family Therapy* 7: 441–52.

———. 1982a. Personal authority via the termination of the intergenerational hierarchy boundary, part 2: The consultation process and the therapeutic method. *Journal of Marriage and Family Therapy* 8: 223–37.

———. 1982b. Personal authority via the termination of the intergenerational hierarchy boundary, part 3: Personal authority defined and the power of play in the change process. *Journal of Marriage and Family Therapy* 8: 309–23.

———, and Bray, J. H. 1988. Family development and change across the generations: An intergenerational perspective. In C. J. Falicov, ed. *Family Transitions*. New York: Guilford Press. 357–84.

Young-Eisendrath, P. 1984. *Hags and Heroes: A Feminist Approach to Jungian Psychotherapy with Couples*. Toronto: Inner City Books.

***Terrill L. Gibson**, Ph.D., is a pastoral psychotherapist and Diploma Jungian Analyst, and a member of Jungian Analysts-North Pacific as well as the International Association for Analytical Psychology. He lectures and writes extensively on the general theme of the relationship of spirituality and psychotherapy. He is an Approved Supervisor with the American Association for Marriage and Family Therapy.*

Toward a Jungian Analysis and Treatment of Systems with Emphasis on Individuation in Relationship

Laura S. Dodson, M.S.W., Ph.D.

Introduction

The implications of Jung's transpersonal psychology were revolutionary in their time. Today they are on the cutting edge of systems thinking in many fields, from biology and chemistry to psychology and the understanding of culture. Jung explored the universe as a total system, of which the individual psyche is but one part of the greater dance.[1] As the first transpersonal psychologist, Jung's genius lay in his exploration of transpersonal energy systems, which have existed since before time and which impact every individual. These energy systems he called "archetypes." Jung's work focused in large part on the intrapsychic system and its interplay with the archetypal system.

Jung saw the symbols in cultures as "bridges" between the individual and the archetype. Archetypes are never fully knowable, but images and symbols as products of the psyche, wondrously full of many levels of meaning that move toward the numinous. They are manifest not only in the dreams of our inner life, but also in collective symbols in all cultures, symbols that are found in rites, rituals, customs, myths, and fairy tales. Study of these collective symbols took Jung into a third systems area, that of culture.

Jung's in-depth study of these three systems—archetypal, intrapsychic, and cultural—as well as his work on intimate and parent/child relationships, provide a rich base both for the development of a systems psychology theory and for the treatment of human systems on all levels. This chapter and this book as a whole are focused on applying and further expanding Jungian psychology, often referred to as "depth psychology," toward the understanding and treatment of couple and family systems.

In the ensuing section of this chapter I first describe some of Jung's basic concepts that set a foundation for the development of a combined depth/systems psychology. The second section of the chapter focuses on archetypes impacting intimate relationships and this is followed, in the third section, by a discussion which sets the system of intimacy in the context of a myriad of systems in which it lives. In my fourth and final section, I discuss a way in which we might view the process of transformation or change within all human systems. This is offered as a contribution toward what I see as an emerging field: Jungian analysis and therapy for human systems on all levels.

I. Jung's Cornerstone Ideas Toward Building a Depth/Systems Psychology

Jung's psychology, a psychology focused on growth rather than illness, has as its key concern the natural drive to develop, "unfold," or actualize the self within. That process, which Jung called "individuation," involves a transpersonal process of the self within as it relates to the central archetype, the Self or Great Self. In Jung's view, the Self is the great archetype; existing apriori, it is an aspect of the divine.

Key in Jungian thought, and in the work of Virginia Satir as well, is the respect, even awe, with which another individual is met in the process of psychotherapy. There is no energetic split between the healer and the wounded. The attitude of the therapist is: we are all on a common human journey. The "wounded/healer" is one archetypal energy, not split in the therapy room with the therapist as healer and the client as wounded. Both aspects are honored in each person, allowing for a partnership of mutual respect in the healing process.

Energy is another key concept in Jungian thought. Energy also exists *a priori* and is a force present in all systems. More akin to new physics than to Freud, Jung viewed the world as a total system. Energies of all systems interplay with and impact on one another, and these energies can transform systems. All systems are in a process of evolution and change. In the process of individuation, the psyche is impacted not only from *within* (by the energy of the libido, repressed material, and early childhood life experiences, as Freudian-based psychology embraces), but also from *without* (by archetypal energies).

Jung coined the word "synchronicity," referring to those moments in life when there is a meeting between the energy of human systems and that of the archetypes. In those moments there is a sense of harmony, oneness, light, numinosity. Jung's recognition of these moments invested psychology with a sense of the awe and mystery of life, and placed intrapsychic processes in a perspective with all systems.

Another word coined by Jung is "complex," which describes split-off autonomous energy, fragments of the psyche that behave as independent energy systems—e.g., when a person behaves as if "beside themselves." The split occurs in relation to personal trauma and/or family or cultural norms, or perhaps even karma or destiny. Jung's psychology is not one of "solving problems," but one of "transforming energy" blocked in complexes, so that the natural flow of energy can move toward individuation.

Much of Jung's work, following the formulation of his theories of energy, individuation, archetypes, and complexes, was an exploration of how energy systems interplay. In his lifetime, he focused mainly on the system of the individual psyche, its treatment, and his theory of archetypal systems. The systems between the individual and archetypes—intimate relationships (marriage), family systems, genealogy, and cultural systems—are discussed throughout the *Collected Works*, but not with a comprehensive approach to systems analysis and treatment. I am confident that Jung never intended the development of his theories and their application to end with his lifetime. His rich works provide a foundation, upon which others can build a depth psychology approach to analysis and treatment of systems.

The inevitable rise and fall of nations, as espoused by Arnold Toynbee, is brought into question when Jung's concept of transformation is applied to national and cultural systems. Can systems on this scale evolve or individuate? Must nations literally die in order to change, or might the "death" be merely a transformation on deeper archetypal and symbolic levels, thus changing the system's functioning?

An individual depth psychology makes us more aware of what we ourselves project outward. A systems psychology enriches us further with an awareness of what is also projected onto us by our families, geneology, cultural unconscious and the unconscious of the world—as well as how these interplay. A combination of systems therapy and depth psychology offers a more complete picture of psyche in systems. One can see more clearly, not only into personal complexes but also into personal family, genealogy, and all human systems. The inclusion of these matters in psychotherapy moves us toward a sense of compassion for all humankind, a sense of world citizenship. Consciousness of the interplay of all systems assists us in taking on the task of standing on the shoulders of generations before us, to do our part in the evolution of consciousness.

The impact of systems upon systems opens the question of individuals' inheriting psychological aspects from ancestors (or having access to their energy systems by means other than environment or biological inheritance). It raises the question of destiny and its relationship to will. In what follows, (sections II., III., IV. of this chapter) I will focus on 1) various archetypes that impact intimate relationships, 2) other human systems that impact intimate relationships, and 3) a process of transformational change applicable to individual, couple, and cultural systems. A study of the impact of systems upon systems move us to a psychology that can step off the planet, move beyond time and space, and look at the big show, bringing these dimensions and consciousness to efforts to find healing of pain of the moment in the office.

II. Archetypes in Intimate Relationships

It is often such a relief for individuals, couples, and families in psychotherapy to see their personal concerns mirrored in myth and folktales throughout history. They come to see their journeys toward individuation and healthy relationships as not unlike other persons' struggles throughout time. Their struggles, in addition to their family history and childhood traumas, are often related to archetypal shifts in their culture today, or in the world as a whole. In this way, individuals, couples, and families can recognize their kinship to humanity. The result is less guilt, shame, and fear, as well as an increased sense of empathy and compassion for the self and others. Archetypal energies often push and pull us around until we become more conscious of these energies and how they connect with our personal, couple, and family dramas. What follows is a discussion of some archetypal energies that affect couple life.

Individuation as the Key Archetypal Process in Intimacy

The self emerges on the foundation of a "good enough" parent-child relationship, and within other relationships that repair or build what was damaged or absent in the parent-child relationship. Jung's concept of marriage as a psychological relationship recognizes marriage itself as one vessel which can contribute to the birth-to-death process of individuation and the healing of childhood wounds. In the desire to set a "theater" of life for the unfolding of the self, we create dramas in which to live our lives. These dramas push the edges of our growth and create opportunities to develop the dark or unrealized sides of ourselves. I know of no other theater that gives more of these opportunities than intimate relationships.

When the container of the relationship is a basically healthy system, we can find the support and mirroring that allows the dark or under-developed sides of the self to emerge and be more integrated into conscious life. A "lethal" potential is also present. Intimate relationships hold the possibility that the individuals involved may become locked into lower levels of functioning, establishing a status quo that is similar in many ways to the dysfunctional aspects of the family systems in the families of origin of those involved. We settle in as if on a bed of nails; it is not necessarily comfortable, but familiarity brings, at least for a time, a false sense of safety. The individuation process has temporarily gone to sleep and functioning is in "automatic gear."

Falling In Love: The First Archetypal Experience in Intimacy

When one falls in love "at first sight," so to speak, Cupid smites, Aphrodite charms. The experience is an ultimate in projection of aspects of the self. It is as if such compelling energy pulls us into a drama in which we can meet shadows, and potentially live on the edge of our growth. The intensity of "falling in love" inevitably moves at some point to its opposite. We must fall out of love, and experience betrayals which are inevitable, for the loved one is obviously not (or at least not only or fully) that which is projected. Projection and reclaiming projections is a normal process, in which lies an opportunity for the relationship to become an arena for individuation.

A couple's most vulnerable time is that time after falling in love, when they find that the projections do not hold. Courage, trust, and understanding of what is happening are needed to move to the next step in a growth-enhancing way.

Marriage as Archetype

Marriage, symbolizing the union of opposites of male and female, is one possible arena to which one may be drawn or elected to meet the opposites within. Other possible arenas for individuation are priesthood or convent, immersion in one's work, etc. Adolf Guggenbühl-Craig, a Jungian analyst, warns that marriage is not the theater for everyone's individuation, though culture sometimes pressures one into feeling it is the only or the best, and that without it one has "failed" (1977, 36).

Whatever theater our unconscious elects, it tends to be one that meets us on the edges of our growth. The theater itself will contain both a potential for falling deeper into one's complexes and a potential for growing beyond these energy blocks. Couples can be in a trance state, stagnated by the archetype of marriage: an externally directed system of behaviors supported by the culture, adopted by the ego, but not necessarily related to the self. These are the relationships which, when the psyche can no longer tolerate the deadness, find themselves in the psychotherapist's office or in divorce court. Fear related to old wounds and ignorance affects the potential of marriage as a vessel for growth, and tragedy too often ensues.

An example is Ted and Jean. After their initial falling in love, patterns developed between them that allowed them to continue in their childhood defenses and complexes, and to bask in the complexes of the family and the culture as if in a stupor or a trance. It was often difficult for them to differentiate wife from mother or husband from father. Seeing the "other" and the self was difficult. The dysfunctional patterns that they evolved offered some comfort and security. This painful state was masked for years; it complied with the expectations of their cultural system. Jean was a "perfect wife and mother," while Ted fulfilled his role as a "hero" in the world.

In some sense, the couple had the experience of "riding high" on role fulfillment and actualization of some aspects of their personalities. In this was camouflaged their defenses against the injured self. Between them, they created a system in which each could "fall asleep" to protect those areas in each of their psyches that were tender and vulnerable. Ted and Jean were enshrouded by the archetype of marriage itself. To the outside world, at least at a glance, they looked like the perfect married couple, until Ted began an affair and after several years Jean caught him and left him in a rage. The form of marriage could no longer sustain this couple. The false self could no longer perform and the true self cried out for space in this world. The crisis was an opportunity to break the trance state of the archetype of marriage.

The Archetype of the Wounded Child

One of Jung's greatest contributions to work with couple and family systems is his study of the great mother and the child archetypes (1951, par. 81–112), and his development of the archetypal theme of abandonment. In referring to Jung's work on these issues, Joseph Wheelwright called Jung the first object relations therapist (1982, 8). Jung saw the personal mother as omnipresent in the psyche of the child, and marked the profundity of abandonment wounds of early childhood as key to functioning throughout life. From this first "intimate" relationship, object relations, or relationship to other, is learned; the pattern of this first experience is a major factor in mate choice and ways of relating to one's mate, particularly for those persons with severe early wounding.

Most of us are in a state of unconsciousness when we enter a commitment to intimacy. We are unconscious of our inner wounded child's desire to find a home, a family, and new openings for the healing of early wounds. This longing, as with Ted and Jean, is kept secret. They were unconscious of it; when it moved into consciousness, it was a source of shame, embarrassment, and rage.

The degree of unconsciousness of their own and the other's wounded child, and the intensity of the early woundings, increases the potential of the wounded child archetype overcoming the marriage. Suddenly, into the home of two people—made four by the projection of the female part of the man onto the woman, and the male part of the woman onto the man, made six or eight by projection of parents onto mates—come the autonomous personalities of two wounded children, home hopefully to rest and nest! If the experience of betrayal has not already occured, it most certainly will. When the wounded child of the past steps out and is not recognized, it again is abandoned. The childhood wound is re-experienced at the hand of the loved one; most frequently, neither partner knows what hit them.

The ever-present themes of attachment and separation in childhood development retain their potency throughout life. The need for bonding also exists throughout life. The paradox of separate and related is always present in intimacy, and is as much the theme of marriage as it is of childhood and adolescence.

Shadow as Archetype in Intimacy

The creative potential for growth was also present in Ted and Jean's marriage. As we worked together, we could document the times in the history of their marriage when creativity attempted to break through the archetypal hold on the marriage. Jean often felt that she wanted to develop herself, to return to school, to expand her creativity. Her urge for development would reject the projection Ted had on her (and that she received as part of her identity). It would disturb the equilibrium in the marriage, a frightening concern for her sense of self—and his as well. To become conscious of shadow aspects of herself was terrifying to Jean. Marriage gave her a place to hide. She would say, "I just wanted to be home and support Ted and the children, be here when they come home, etc. He was my hero." Her fear of her own hero was shadowed or under-developed, and projected onto the marriage. Ted carried it for her, which contributed to his false sense of self-identity and protected him from facing shadowed or under-developed aspects of himself. Ted did not need to look at his fear of intimacy, rooted in repeated parent and step-parent loss, as long as he could busy himself in work and carry Jean's hero projection.

Their marriage became one of the mother archetype being lived out by Jean, with some aspects of *puella* (eternal girl) and lover also present in the marriage. Ted was engulfed by the archetype of the hero. As this system became more rigid, his *puer* (eternal boy) found its expression with an extramarital relationship. As the mother archetype dominated Jean's life, other aspects of a woman's self, the wise woman or medium, and the Amazon or heroine, as well as the more mature lover, remained in shadow in Jean's psyche (DeCastillejo 1973, 44–64). For Ted, the father and the wise man remained in the unconscious, the *puer* and hero in the foreground. This marriage system maintained a balance that was taut and increasingly inflexible. The vessel of the marriage, we could say, became polluted. It could not hold two persons as they individuated, but became instead a repository of unclaimed parts of the self and a defense against unrealized or shadow parts of the self. As such, its malfunctioning also contributed to blocks in the individuation of their children.

Movement Toward the Dynamic Archetype of Nuptial *Coniunctio*

Jung's description of *coniunctio* (1954a, par. 654–789) is a powerful model for intimacy in relationships. *Coniunctio* for inner marriage with the self is the deepest drive we have. For Jung, the process of developing this internal relationship is an intense and exciting dynamic in life, the core of the individuation process.

Of course, no one marries or has children in order to have pain or feel imprisoned, or contribute to those feelings in another. Our yearning to allow ourselves to be at one with another battles with the fear of destroying the fragile sense of self we may have barely managed to create. From this fear and ignorance of how to evolve something better, and from the reinforcement of dysfunctional systems that move in upon us from family of origin, genealogy, and culture, limiting and archetypally possessed systems evolve. It is also possible that in intimacy, when we can return to our vulnerability and feel for the most part safe to be with another in that state, we can find a recovery of the being that we lost or never achieved. In this vulnerability is the paradox of strength to heal and grow.

Nuptial *coniunctio* is a dynamic interpersonal archetypal process in which individuation occurs. As opposed to a stagnant archetypal possession, in the archetype of nuptial *coniunctio* the systems within and between the individuals are in constant change. Change is the only certainty. Life is a process, not a stagnant outcome. The institution of marriage simply lends an outer form to give some order to the process of movement toward union of opposites within and without (Jung 1954a, par. 88). The dynamic process connotes a vessel of trust in which persons can be vulnerable. It offers a place for potential recovery of early wounding, and development of the self.

At midlife, the under-developed aspects of Ted and Jean cried out to be released from the lethal prison they had unconsciously evolved in their marriage. To address the issue of developing the self would disturb not only their inner life and their marriage, but systems at every level, including marriage, family, extended family, work, cultural systems, and archetypal systems. They struggled. T. S. Eliot describes this state in his poem, "The Love Song of J. Alfred Prufrock":

> And indeed there will be time
> To wonder, "Do I dare?" and, "Do I dare?"
> Time to turn back and descend the stair,
> With a bald spot in the middle of my hair—
> . . . .
> Do I dare
> Disturb the universe?
> In a minute there is time
> For decisions and revisions which a minute will reverse.
> . . . .
> And the afternoon, the evening, sleeps so peacefully!
> Smoothed by long fingers,
> Asleep . . . tired . . . or it malingers,
> Stretched on the floor, here beside you and me.
> Should I, after tea and cakes and ices,
> Have the strength to force the moment to its crisis?
> But though I have wept and fasted, wept and prayed,
> Though I have seen my head [grown slightly bald] brought in upon
> a platter,
> I am no prophet—and here's no great matter;
> I have seen the moment of my greatness flicker,
> And I have seen the eternal Footman hold my coat, and snicker,
> And in short, I was afraid. (ll. 37–40, 45–48, 75–86)

Ted once described the price his soul paid in his thirty-year, ideal-to-the-American-world marriage: "I knew what suit I would wear every Monday, Tuesday, etc. I knew what I would do every day. I felt stagnated and depressed. I was glad in a way that she caught me in my affair. In a strange way I am more alive now than I have been for years." The price for the equilibrium that allowed a temporary repose was a certain ritualistic quality to life, in time a lessening of creative energy, and eventually stagnation, repression, and depression.

Crisis in intimacy can be seen as the cry of the psyche to individuate and to break the complexes in the individuals and the couple system. Crisis contains the seed of an opportunity for growth. When much of the partner's inner turmoil is projected on and acted out in the relationship, ending the relationship can seem like the only way to end the pain. The task of the therapist becomes that of enhancing safety while unveiling the inner systems of both partners (their complexes and early wounds) and the system between them, and to make these systems and how they intertwine more conscious. These systems must be placed in the context of familial, genealogical, cultural, and archetypal systems in order to complete a treatment both in depth psychology and systems analysis. Then, the possibility of the marriage becoming a vessel for individuation is enhanced, and a more conscious decision can be made as to whether the couple will choose the task of building a growth-enhancing system in their marriage, fall back asleep, or dissolve the marriage.

A marriage works (has a growth or creative potential) if one opens oneself to exactly that which one would never ask for otherwise. It is only through rubbing oneself sore and losing oneself that one is able to learn about oneself, God, and the world. Like every soteriological pathway, that of marriage is hard and painful (Guggenbühl-Craig, 1977, 45).

In intimate relationships, the dynamic archetypal process of *coniunctio* is enlivened when courage and curiosity dominate over fear, when humility, vulnerability, and forgiveness allow one to admit and mourn human frailty and move on rather than protect or project it. The goal, though never fully achievable, is for each partner to meet self within and to meet that in the other. This is achieved in the fire of the alchemical vessel of marriage itself, where the active theater kindles projections, and a "healthy enough process" is achieved to allow for reclaiming of projections and working them through within, in a holding, caring, vessel of the relationship and with increasing trust in the process of wounding and healing that the two have entered.

As Jung explicitly states, the individuation process is made up of struggles between the ego and the unconscious, each at once having its way, as much as we can stand; between the two, as between a hammer and an anvil the individual is made (1963, par. 521–3). Yet another hammer and anvil for individuation exists in intimate relationships and in the family. There, as one rubs up against shadows and projections, and in the process differentiates the self, individuation and intimacy have a keen opportunity.

In her chapter in this book, Polly Young-Eisendrath discusses practical details in the development of a healthy relationship in terms of a therapy process that moves from communication to the depth of the psyche. Ann Ulanov's chapter discusses into more depth *coniunctio* in marriage. I continue here to set a broader context of the myriad of energy systems in which our intimate relationship lives, systems that greatly impact intimacy.

III. Other Human Systems Which Impact Intimate Relationships

Intimate relationships, with all their archetypal pulls, do not exist only in the arena of self-couple archetype systems. Family, genealogical, and cultural systems as well as archetypal shifts in the world today also greatly impact our intimate relationships. Personal and couples issues cannot be viewed or treated as personal problems alone; rather, they exist in the myriad of systems upon systems, and can reflect complexes in all systems external to and including the personal psyche.

Jung emphasized connection of the self to the Great Self. I propose that between these two systems there are other human systems that impact this connection (see Graph, p. 43). Depending on their health, all systems between the individual and the archetypal Self can be conduits or blocks to the connection of the self with the archetypal Self. How then to increase the health of all these systems becomes a critical goal of the individuation process. How can Jungian analysis develop a psychology of and treatment approach to this myriad of systems?

Expanding Jung's thinking about the individuation process in the human psyche, we could say that all human systems are drawn toward the process of individuating not only each person, but also couple systems, family systems, even cultures. Applying Jung's term, individuation, to these systems allows us to examine their relative health or individuation, and gives us a base for describing their process of change. Virginia Satir offers a list of component parts within all human systems: a) the persons involved, b) the patterns of behavior or rules of the systems, c) the context, d) the balance or flexibility, and e) the price and payoff for the system to operate (1991, 177–78). Her concept, echoes Kenneth Boulding, who offers a way in which to study and "unveil" human systems (1985, 11). Jungian psychology approaches systems analysis through dreams, symbols, myths and metaphors. By applying Satir's systems analysis and Jungian

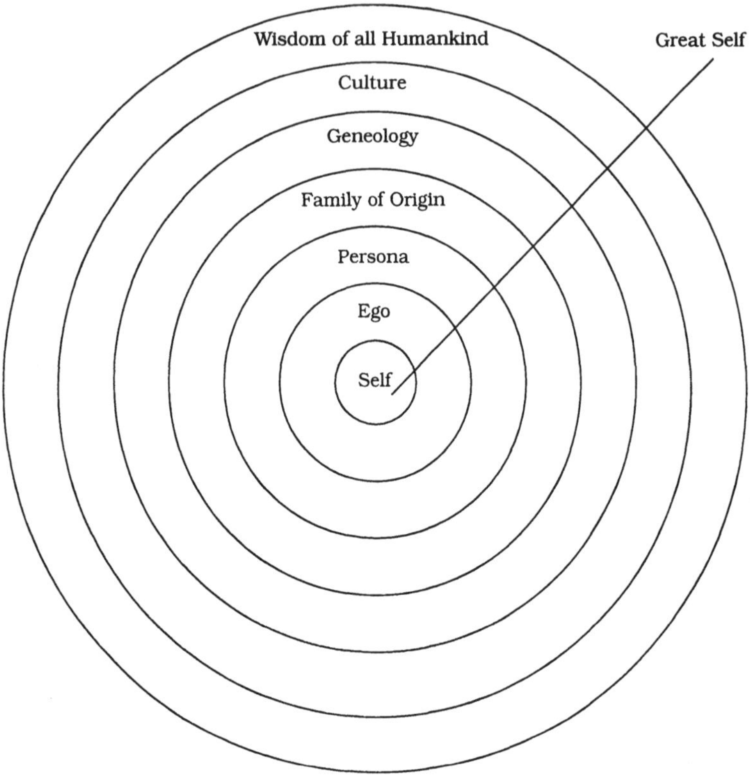

Graph. Human Systems

depth psychology, analysis can work toward systems change at the roots of the issues, while at the same time responding to the issues immediately at hand.

The Family and Genealogical System

Unresolved and unconscious issues from one's family of origin and even one's genealogical family come into marriage. Mother and father are projected onto mate, and these projections must be withdrawn before two individuals can begin to move toward a meeting of the self within and the self within the other. These also will be re-enacted in the creation of one's own family system. I will not delve here into the many aspects of Jungian psychology as it relates to family and genealogy. Some of this is covered in other chapters, other aspects are best saved for later books. Here I would like to underscore the importance of systems analysis coupled with depth personal analysis.

An expansion of Jung's ideas enriches the personal introspective search, connecting one with archetypes through myth. Jungian analysis of the myths of family relationships—such as "The Handless Maiden," "Hansel and Gretel," "Snow White," "Iron John," etc.—symbolically illuminate various aspects of abandonment, betrayal, problems of projection, projective identification, sacrifice of the self, etc., rooted in family life. Further, Jung suggests that these complexes, while personal in nature and rooted in family of origin, are also a part of energy systems greater than the individual and his/her family. They may have a genealogical as well as an archetypal core. As I see it, intertwining analysis of systems on all levels is essential to healing in depth.

Archetypal Shifts in Today's World

In 1958, in his essay on UFOs, Jung predicted the emergence of the archetype of the self as we approach the year 2000 (1958, par. 589–824). He saw the spherical flying objects projected onto the skies as symbols of wholeness, or the archetypal self. Because the phenomena occurred in over forty nations, Jung saw them as evidence of a collective issue for all the world, signaling a major shift in the psyche of all humankind. Since Jung was concerned about the dangers of persons being "swallowed up" by emerging archetypal energy when one is unconscious of what is emerging (and therefore unprepared to meet that energy), in his essays he warned people to get ready for the disruption of the psyche caused by archetypal shifts, and to meet these shifts with an ego strong enough to integrate them into consciousness. In this way the shifts can be opportunities for increased consciousness and individuation.

Is what Jung predicted really happening? Is a greater union of the masculine/feminine energy, within and without, coming upon us? I believe so. In the thirty-eight years since Jung's prediction, shifts have occurred in both the masculine and feminine archetypes as well as in the child archetype. These shifts are erupting in our personal lives, our marriages, and our families in such a way that we cannot behave as we once did. We see that such shifts have their effects on cultures as well, as can be seen with the fall of the iron curtain. It is as if some feminine spiritual aspects were deepened during oppression behind the iron curtain, where the scientific and industrial revolution had little detracting impact on inner life. Now, these energies are unleashed and are impacting western cultures. Cultures with a more feminine-dominant (*yin*) energy are moving toward integrating masculine (*yang*) energy, and vice versa. Old patterns, patterns that tell us how we should be, are disrupted on all levels. The old ego-consciousness must shift to make way for new movement in the development of the self, and a new level of consciousness of the ego/self axis must evolve. We are in the liminal stage of this archetypal change—unable to return to the old, but not yet evolved into new ways of being.

Historically, America has been dominated by the archetypal stance of men as heroes. This archetype was the culmination of three thousand years of culture increasingly dominated by *yang* energy. The archetype served its purpose; the "rugged individual" was central to the fabric of the American dream. We denied pain, human neediness, and human limitations to charge forth to meet the challenges of conquering a new land. The goal was attained, in a sense, but as is the case with any archetypal possession, we pay a price, and now stand in need of correction on all levels: personal, familial, and cultural.

We become more conscious of the price we have paid when we try to integrate suppressed parts of the self. We become aware that the child and the feminine were repressed on the rugged individual journey, and that men were boxed in containers too small for the healthy development of their psyches. We can see unintegrated parts of the self contained in women, in children, and in minorities, and in the repressed aspect of men.

Blacks and women were the first to demand release from their confinement; the women's movement and the Black Power movement emerged as collective carriers of this archetypal shift. Such movements created a great deal of energy; as with all dramatic shifts in consciousness, they carry their share of projection, denial, over-identification, and other coping mechanisms. In the face of the emerging energy, such coping mechanisms are a natural part of collective shifts in consciousness. The women's movement had its extreme pendulum swing expressed by raging, angry women, and is now experiencing a corrective. Now, men are seen less as the enemy and more as fellow human beings in need of major shifts in their psyche as well. There is progress in the movement, away from blame and toward more freedom in roles and self-development.

The men's movement now focuses on shedding or integrating some of the hero/rugged individual archetypal energy with other parts of the self. Initially it fell into over-identification with the emerging feminine energy; we saw men become more aware of feminine characteristics like softness, holding, reflecting. Many persons have become lost, some into drugs, many suffered a lack of focus. Some men denied this feminine energy, and attempted to restore the old order. Now there is more evidence that men are integrating the shadow aspects of themselves and expanding their role possibilities in the culture. We are moving toward a realization of the deeper aspects of what it means to integrate masculine and feminine, *yin* and *yang*, anima and animus, and move toward development of cultural forms that facilitate this shift.

In the last several years, the "adult children" movement has developed, signaling a shift in the last of the three major archetypes of masculine, feminine, child. The Alcoholics Anonymous movement has recognized the wounded child and affirmed it, but over-identification with the child archetype has been part of the inevitable pendulum swing as we seek to heal this archetype. The wounded child is an archetypal shadow to the American culture. The wounded child is our new hero in a sense. The actual child and the wounded child archetype now carry the seeds for personal and cultural healing. The dark side of this emerging energy is that the images of ourselves as wounded are a new place in which to be stuck, e.g., if we catch the pendulum swing away from the silent, repressed child, but remain at the other extreme position, that of the raging child, we remain bound by the wounded child archetype.

During the dominance of the myth of the rugged individual, the actual child had the extraordinary burden of carrying the hurt and rejected inner child for the parent who unconsciously projected his or her own woundedness onto their child. The parent then rejected the actual child by failing too often to see the child as a real person. In the first half of this century, the child was generally portrayed as innocent and joyful, expected to appreciate authority and to be subordinate to adults. A culture of "children are to be seen, and not heard" existed. Then we became a culture of idealizing, but at the same time depersonalized children. They were like Hummel figurines in much of the larger culture's minds, or they were gradually moved to the still-idealized but somewhat more human Norman Rockwell portraits on the front of *The Saturday Evening Post*. In any case, they were a repository for unclaimed aspects of the child in the adults.

The actual child of today is changing and, as changes go, it has moved to its opposite extreme by the broad swing of the pendulum. The actual child is cutting loose to rage. We see it in increased use of firearms for random murder on the part of children. We see a lack of focus in the lives of our children; they sense that there is no meaning to life.

The "adult child" too is enraged, feeling that he or she is entitled to reparation. These newly-awakened children in our culture now point the finger at their abusers, revealing secrets and confronting issues. This conscious anger and rage is an important step in the evolution toward healing, both for the child within each of us and for the child archetype in the culture—important in that it moves toward all aspects of the child having a voice, and toward wholeness of the child archetype with all its parts.

However, as with the women's movement and the Black movement, this and all movements must continue beyond the polarity of abused/abuser, innocent/blamed, victim/perpetrator. Without continued growth in consciousness, the pendulum swing can become yet another rigid stance. The goal is manifestations of all aspects of the archetype. Systems within the individual psyche and in the cultural run the risk of possession by a new aspect of the archetypal child, that of demonic innocence.

All of these archetypal shifts greatly affect couple and family life. Awareness of them can assist couples and families to see their personal pain as a part of a larger transformation in culture. Empathy for self and other is increased, empowering the individual to contribute not only to personal and family change, but also to shifts in consciousness in larger systems.

IV. Toward a Process of Transformational Change in Human Systems

There are, I believe, common processes that describe healthy transformation in all human systems, from the personal psyche to systems relationships of intimacy and family, and including genealogical systems and cultural systems. Of course, transformation is a process that cannot be canned, or made to happen, but we can move toward it.

At the risk of seeming reductive, but in an effort to "get a

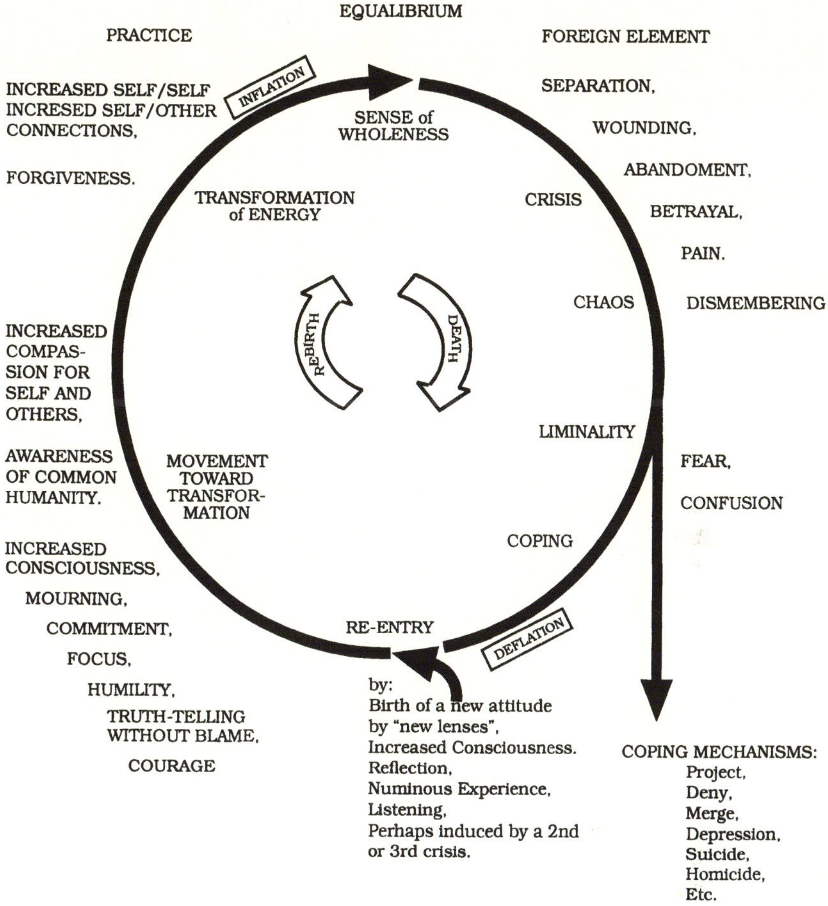

Chart. Human Transformation and Change

handle" on the process of growth and change, I attempt here to describe stages in the process of transformation in human systems. My chart (above) was inspired in part by Edward Edinger's "Psychic Life Cycle" (1972, 41). It gives an outline of movement toward transformation. I will walk through it three times, once in relation to individual transformation, once in relation to couple and family transformation, and lastly, in relation to cultural transformation.

A. Beginning at the top of the chart and moving right, we see the fetus or infant exposed to its first interruption of well-being. There are no perfect parents. Abandonment to some degree is a phenomenon of all human life. Perhaps the first betrayal is even conception itself, where we are separated from universal energies and encapsulated in a body. Or maybe the first inevitable separation or abandonment is birth, when we are cast out of the womb. Abandonments and betrayals come not only from external sources, but also from abandonment of the self. Separation from aspects of the self is an essential process in the development of the first complex, the ego. Development of the ego is necessary for adapting to and living in the world, and thus it is a necessary abandonment of self. In time, as individuation occurs, the ego can become subservient to the self. As such the ego is an instrument of the self rather than a split-off complex.

We are thrown into chaos and pain, and even, at times, into the agonizing sense of dismemberment, abandonment, and betrayal (two o'clock position on the chart). Our equilibrium disrupted by these crises; we are betwixt and between, in limbo; our universe is upset. As young children, even as infants, despite our limited experience of life and limited tools for coping, we must find ways to deal with this pain and make new order out of the chaos (four o'clock on chart).

To stabilize the ego, we develop coping mechanisms or defenses against the pain. From our families, we learn "acceptable" defense patterns that can help us tolerate stress. We may attempt to restore the old order, and/or deny that anything has happened; we may become depressed, self-blaming, rageful to others, decide not to trust again, attempt to merge with a nurturing object, or miss out on ego development. We may feel suicidal or homicidal (scc chart, five o'clock position).

In time we can hope that another crisis—some numinous or positive experience of life, will occur to jolt us, wake us, and create an opportunity for growth. And, we can hope that it will come at a time when we feel the ego strength and outer life stability to allow us to take the courage we need in order to move toward healing (seven and eight o'clock positions).

Shifts occurring in the archetypal child offer a specific example with which to describe the process of change. Because of the nature of the child itself, it is very easy for the child to remain stuck in a repetitive manner at the point on the diagram of attempted reentry from the defensive position, and then be unable to move around to the left side of the circle past the five o'clock position. This issue has to do with the extraordinary vulnerability of the child who, by its very nature, can perceive only one thing to be true at a time. For the child with pre-verbal wounding, to move toward duplicity and contain opposites is particularly difficult. The following are steps at the point of reentry which are particularly characteristic of those with early wounding.

1. In the transformation process, "adult children" first experience rage, hurt, insult, vulnerability, and even hate, which swallows them in its agony. This is not the rage or projection described as "coping mechanisms" on the chart. It has a pregnant-like quality as contrasted to a stagnant quality. The adult child feels again the abandonment, betrayal, and abuse as he/she re-experiences it, rages about it, and feels righteous indignation about it.

2. It is quite possible to become stuck in this stage, and to come to enjoy the innocence of this position and the rage that protects that innocence. A moralistic stance can develop. The "adult children's movement" has often been stuck here. What is needed, once consciousness of early wounding is gained, is seeing the connection to present pain, and gaining the ability to differentiate and relate it to present pain in the self and in one's intimate relations. Then the individual or each partner in the relationship can begin to cope with present distress, and unload the unconscious "baggage" of the past. The adult can come to see that when old abandonment wounds are tapped in the marriage, their fear of their very survival, which they felt as a child, has been re-invoked. Such danger need not be present in their intimate relationship, as many more creative possibilities can be learned with which to deal with and transform the pain than ever were possible in their more helpless and dependent state as children. Consciousness and a safe environment in therapy that is tested over and over again is a key to transformation of these wounds, wounds so lethal to intimacy.

Movement toward such a transformation is a difficult art even in psychotherapy. The art is enriched not only by Jung's work on the wounded child, but also by object relations theory and self psychology. Jung's unique contribution to healing on this level is the self related to the Great Self, a concept often seen by object relations theorists as a denial of the state of abandonment. To a Jungian, abandonment must still be worked through, but a state of connection with the "great mother" archetype, in the absence of the real mother, is present in the dreams and images of the young child who is wounded. This archetypal parent can sustain the frail inner child as the adult gropes to move past these wounds. It gives the person with early wounding an opposite experience in maturing to that of those not so wounded. They first contact the transpersonal parent and then must learn to relate to human beings, whereas in more normal development, a person would relate to actual parents as god-like figures, then see their frailty. Then, as a separate identity evolves further later in life, a connection with the transpersonal occurs.

3. If sufficient safety occurs for the child on a personal and/or collective level (achieved through appropriate boundaries and a nurturing container in the present), the child or adult child moves toward duplicity, or the ability to hold opposites in the psyche (example: good mother, bad mother). In this stage, wounded children experience themselves as both the abused and the abuser, the betrayed and the betrayer, the demonic innocent. This movement toward duplicity is essential for healing. Once the child has developed to the point of containing, even in fleeting moments, the possibility of duplicity, then entry to the second half of the circle on the chart occurs, and growth can continue.

The individual can then move to truth-telling without blame, and mourning for what has been or has not been (seven o'clock position on the chart). It is then that a person must be steadfast and have an ego strong enough as he/she goes around the circle of transformation to meet new emerging issues. As with all persons on this common human journey, we move ahead with responsibility and commitment to ourselves and to life itself. We move toward an awareness that our lot is part of being human, part of life's process of wounding and healing; we are a part of a journey common to all humankind. In the process of healing and growth, we feel compassion for ourselves and others, and more acceptance of what is (eight and nine o'clock positions on the chart). The capacity for forgiveness may "come upon us." It is a gift of grace. We cannot choose it, but we can move toward it by the other aspects of healing described on the chart (see seven through ten o'clock positions). Then, moving to the eleven and twelve o'clock positions, we feel once again more deeply connected to ourselves and to others. Energy is transformed (see inside circle on chart, eleven o'clock position) and we again feel a sense of wholeness.

B. A couple or family's journey of transformation and change can be traced in this chart, also. Each partner, in his or her own childhood, has learned ways of dealing with abandonment and betrayal. When the betrayals which are inevitable in relationship occur, the earlier learned coping mechanisms extend to the marriage relationship as defenses to protect against old wounds, resulting in fear of the self and of intimacy. Members of the couple and family system are ready targets for projection as a way of coping with present pain as well as original abandonments and betrayals.

Intimacy also brings the possibility of entering into a new vessel in which we try to heal earlier wounds (six o'clock position) and continue individuation. Too frequently, without self-awareness and consciousness of better tools than we had as a child to cope with crisis and chaos, we develop in intimacy a system that operates in a rigid manner, making little room for the development of the self and the relationship. Like a teeter-totter upon which we try to hold a still position of balance, we unconsciously attempt to build a system where we feel safe, though often such efforts to maintain status quo result in falling into an "archetypal trance state." The price of equilibrium is a price to the life and evolution of the soul. A sense of false safety is achieved. Coping mechanisms dominate the relationship (five o'clock position).

When people in intimate relationships or in families hurt one another, old wounds are reopened. This can be viewed as an opportunity for growth, but somehow we must find the inner and outer supports that will enable us to risk connecting with the self within as well as with the other. Only with this kind of support can we gain awareness, assurance, and hope that healing can take place; only then will we have the courage and humility to say we are sorry, to mourn our pain of the past, and to connect and then separate that pain from our pain of the present, and take responsibility for our own growth and limitations. We must gain more curiosity about our similarities and differences, instead of fearing them, and more acceptance of the life process of wounding and healing. We must forgive ourselves and the other, and move into deeper connection with self and the other—over and over again—if our marriages are to become vessels to hold us as we individuate (six to eleven o'clock positions).

C. The chart of human transformation and growth also applies to cultural change. Applied to the United States, in the early days of our country's history, we were in an inflated, idealized state of consciousness. As immigrant, we set out to "conquer" and exploit the new land. Our drive to our goal brought success; we became "number one" among developed nations. We became the benevolent "Big Daddy," and found it hard to comprehend why our control and superiority in giving should anger other nations. We began to fall from our inflated position as we were confronted in jolting ways by our own shadows—in the Black movement, the woman's movement, the war on poverty, and Viet Nam. We felt shame as a nation; we fell into crisis, chaos, and deflation. We fell into a crisis—the loss of the cultural container for our ego identity—and found ourselves betwixt and between, unable to go back to our isolation and hero position and unable to move forward; we found ourselves in a liminality state, in limbo (one o'clock to three-thirty positions). Who are we as men, as women, as children, as family? in our religion? as a nation? All the fundamental questions of identity were being asked.

In an attempt at soothing ourselves, we moved into defense patterns as we escalated the arms race and declared, "We will be Number One" (coping mechanisms, four-thirty position). At times we became depressed at our shortcomings; ashamed to be American, we "threw the baby out with the bathwater." At other times, however, we have taken the courage to see the edges of our growth with optimism, beyond deflation and coping mechanisms, and have moved back on the wheel of transformation (six o'clock position). In a democracy, ideally, there is a built-in process by which a cultural system may be able to correct itself. It allows for the expression of the unconscious as it emerges, a natural corrective which can influence change in the overall culture.

The humility necessary for transformation is difficult for a nation of rugged individualists. We have yet to move into mourning without being lost in guilt or shame. We struggle to move toward recognition of ourselves as a part of a common human journey with all the world, all nations, all cultures. And so we can see what is needed for transformation in our culture as we move around the circle of the chart toward the six o'clock position and beyond. This concept is more akin to the sociologist Victor Turner's description of cultural liminality than to Arnold Toynbee's concept of the rise and fall of nations.

Whether enough people have an ego strong enough to meet the emerging archetypal energies is the determining factor, according to Jung, as to whether or not we will have a third world war. Will literal death be necessary to usher in the transformation of the basic archetypes of male, female, and child?

The entire field of psychology is in a process of change impacted by East meeting West in this time. It is as if the former U.S.S.R. was encapsulated during Stalin's time, its masses isolated from the negative and positive outcome of the scientific revolution, even from aspects of industrialization. This, along with their rich spiritual heritage and communal heritage—and, for the most part, their absence of a Freudian psychology—brings to the evolving field a dimension that can offer us a corrective to rugged individualism, and bring some of the corrective we need. A further expansion that must be mentioned here to gain the whole systems picture is a quote from Kenneth Boulding:

> It would certainly be presumptuous to suppose that systems complexity ended at the level of human race. Just as an ant has very little conception of the human system that may be hovering over it, except perhaps a dim perception of something large and perhaps dangerous, or a dog perceives us as a benign diety and not as another dog, so we may stretch forth intimations of what is beyond us. Certainly our ideas about the transcendent have a profound impact on human and social systems. (1985, 29–30)

Boulding's perception includes for me not only archetypal systems but ecological systems, astrological systems, and many other systems, as yet unknown, that impact human systems. While we divide systems to try to comprehend their parts, we must remember with humility the many known and unknown systems that are all interwoven; harmony or disharmony with them also affects human systems.

Summary

There are definitive Jungian concepts that offer a rich theoretical basis for systems psychology and treatment of systems. These concepts can be applied to treatment of the systems of the personal psyche, the couple, and the family; to understanding the impact of genealogical systems on persons; and to analysis and treat cultural systems. All of these must be viewed in the context of the impact of archetypes on human systems. Further, I have proposed in this chapter a definable process of change or transformation which can assist us in guided transformation of human systems at all levels. Understanding these concepts can enrich the further development of a combined depth/systems psychology, and enrich or amplify the treatment of all human systems.

Note

1. *System* is defined in Webster's *New World Dictionary* (Simon & Schuster, 1980) as "a set or arrangement of things related or connected so as to form unity or organic whole (solar system, school system, etc), chemistry—a group of substances in or approaching equilibrium."

   Defined by Kenneth Boulding and Virginia Satir, all systems have parts and a relationship among the parts, patterns, or "rules" of behavior of the parts, range of flexibility, and a striving for balance or equilibrium.

References

Bellah, R. N. 1985. *Habits of the Heart: Individualism and Commitment in American Life*. Berkeley, CA: University of California Press.

Boulding, K. 1985. *The World as a Total System*. London: Sage Publications.

DeCastillejo, I. C. 1973. *Knowing Woman: A Feminine Psychology*. N.Y.: Harper Colophon.

Dodson, L. S. 1977. *Family Counseling, A Systems Approach*. Muncie, Ind.: Accelerated Development.

———. 1983a. Intertwining Jungian depth psychology and family therapy through use of action techniques. *Journal of Group Psychotherapy, Psychodrama and Sociometry* 35.4.

———. 1983b. Combined analytic and system approaches in working with families. Academy Forum. *Journal of the American Academy of Psychoanalysis*.

———. 1986. An archetypal view of world distress. *Inward Light* Spring, 7–15.

———. 1987. Problems and pitfalls at the crossroads of cultural change. *Inward Light. Spring.*

Edinger, E. F. 1972. *Ego and Archetype*. Baltimore: Penguin.

Eliot, T. S. 1971. *Selected Poems of T. S. Eliot*. San Diego: Harvest. 112–14.

Freud, S. 1961. *Civilization and Its Discontents*. New York: W. W. Norton & Co.

Gordon, L. H. 1993. *Passage to Intimacy*. New York: Simon & Schuster.

Guggenbühl-Craig, A. 1977. *Marriage—Dead or Alive*. Zurich, Switzerland: Spring Publications.

Harman, W. 1988. *Global Mind Change*. Indianapolis: Knowledge Systems Inc.

Hillman, J. 1975. *Loose Ends*. Zurich, Switzerland: Spring Publications.

———. 1981. *The Thought of the Heart and the Soul of the World*. Dallas: Spring Publications.

Jung, C. G. 1951. The psychology of the child archetype. In *CW* 9i: 151–81. Princeton, N.J.: Princeton University Press, 1959.

———. 1954a. The *coniunctio*. *CW* 14, Princeton, N. J.: Princeton University Press, 1963.

———. 1954b. The mother archetype. In *CW* 9i: 81–112, Princeton, N. J.: Princeton University Press, 1959.

———. 1958. Flying saucers: a modern myth of things seen in the skies. In *CW* 10: 311–433. Princeton, N. J.: Princeton University Press, 1964.

Machtiger, H. G. 1985. Perilous beginnings: Loss, abandonment, and transformation. *A Review of Jungian Analysis Abandonment*. Wilmette, Il: Chiron Publications.

Satir, V. Personal notes from her lectures, 1961–1969. Denver, Colorado and Esalen Institute, California.

———. 1988. *The New People Making*. Palo Alto: Science and Behavior Books.

———. 1991. *The Satir Model*. Palo Alto: Science and Behavior Books.

Slipp, S. 1984. *Object Relations: A Dynamic Bridge Between Individual and Family Treatment*. New York: Jason Aronson.

Toynbee, A. 1947. *The Study of History*. In ten vols.

Ulanov, A. 1981. *Receiving Woman*. Philadelphia: Westminster Press.

Wheelwright, J. 1982. *St. George and the Dandelion*. San Francisco: C. G. Jung Institute of San Francisco.

DODSON

Laura S. Dodson, *M.S.W., Ph.D., is a Diplomat Jungian analyst, couple and family therapist. Extensively trained with Virginia Satir, family therapist, and trained in Freudian thought, psychodrama, and gestalt therapy, Laura has practiced psychotherapy for 36 years. She teaches and lectures throughout this country and abroad. Laura has applied her work in Jung and Systems in several eastern European countries, related to recovery from oppression. She is the author of* Family Counseling, A Systems Approach, *and numerous articles.*

Archetypes in Adolescent Development and Psychopathology

Sue Crommelin, L.C.S.W.

Adolescence is the vital developmental stage which lies between puberty and the establishment of one's own household.[1] During this period, adolescents must evolve from being children in a family to being adult members of the societal collective—ready to take their place in the community. Immaturity, with its admixture of defiance and dependence, must be weathered by both youth and family. Winnicott notes that "the only cure for immaturity is the passage of time" (Winnicott 1982, 149). Accordingly, it is important for adults to allow time and space for the immaturity of the adolescent, and to provide the tempered confrontation and limit-setting that the immature and still irresponsible girl or boy must have in order to grow.

Adolescence and Consciousness

Jung attributed a crucial role to adolescence—psychic birth. Psychic birth is the conscious differentiation from one's parents which normally takes place at the time of the eruption of sexuality, i.e., at puberty. Jung claimed that the eruption of sexuality constellates an internal division that has not previously existed in the child, and that this phenomenon is the beginning of the second stage of development. From this point in time, "[e]very problem forces us to greater consciousness and separates us even farther from the unconscious paradise of childhood" (Jung 1931, 751).

Clinging and opposition are major dynamics in adolescence. Jung contended that the source of most adolescent problems is the adolescent's wrenching sense that the demands of life are too harshly putting an end to the dreams of childhood. Thus, Jung asserted that "clinging to the childhood level of consciousness" (Jung, 1931, par. 764) is the common denominator of the problems of youth. "Something in us," he said, "wishes to remain a child, to be unconscious" (Jung 1931, par. 764). Aggression is implicit in the act of growing up and separating from one's parents. By ceasing to view his or her parents through the eyes of a child, the adolescent is discarding archetypal views of both the self and the parents that have become confining. Opposition is thus a central dynamic in adolescent feeling and behavior toward parents and authority. What was formerly containing has now become confining. It may even be perceived to be terrible, smothering, and destructive to the adolescent's emerging individuality. Young people "struggle to establish a personal identity, not to fit into an assigned role, but to go through whatever has to be gone through" (Winnicott 1965, qtd. in Davis & Wallbridge 1981, 82). As a consequence, the adolescent's struggle for self-definition or "to feel real," may sometimes manifest itself in defiant, antisocial, and even violent behavior.

Erich Neumann was the first theorist to apply Jung's ideas of the Self to child and adolescent development (1973; 1976). Neumann conceptualized the development of consciousness as a sequence of archetypal stages. In his view, particular levels of ego development correlate with these archetypal stages. Each successive level of ego development is founded on a specific dominant archetype that holds and structures the ego. At each stage, the Self incarnates itself in an archetype, yet does not become identical to it. The archetype's positive aspect is shown by the attraction toward and interest in the components of the next phase toward which the ego is being driven. Its negative or terrible aspect is manifested as fear of, and clinging to, the phase that is being left behind or transcended.

The first half of life is marked by two decisive developmental crises, each corresponding to what Neumann calls a "dragon fight" (1973, 205). A dragon fight occurs whenever a rebirth or a re-orientation of consciousness becomes necessary. The first developmental crisis deals with the problems of the First Parents and formation of the ego (between the ages of three and five). In this crisis, the child's parents must provide the secondary security of the human world when the ego emerges from the uroboric state of primary union with the mother.[2]

The second dragon fight occurs in puberty, when a new relationship between the ego and the Self emerges. Puberty is "a time of rebirth culminating in the symbolic hero who regenerates himself through fighting the dragon, thus becoming ready for initiation into the larger community" (Neumann 1973, 400–3). Failure in a dragon fight leaves the child immersed in the force-field of the parents:

> To be a mother's darling is a sign of not having accomplished the initial dragon fight which brings infancy to a close. This failure makes entry into school and the world of other children impossible, just as failure in the rites of initiation at puberty [i.e., the second dragon fight] precludes entry into the adult world of men and women." (Neumann 1973, 403)

From this perspective, the developmental task to be accomplished in adolescence is to detach the *archetypal* parents from the *personal* parents. When successfully detached from the personal parents, the archetype of the First Parents is projected onto the larger world outside the family. Projection of the father archetype shapes the adolescent's relation to the figure of master, teacher or leader. The projection of the mother archetype structures one's views of country, community, church, or political movement.

Neumann divided the predominant adolescent syndrome of the dragon fight into four sub-phases. It is noteworthy that Neumann dealt only with males when he described these categories: 1) the son-lover's passive and sweet languishing at the behest of the Great Mother, 2) the struggling lover who is torn by guilt, fear, hate and fascination with the Terrible Mother, 3) the young hero, who wins his battle against the dragon, and 4) the young man who is ready to be initiated as a grown-up member of the collective.

Son-Lover

Adolescents between the ages of twelve and fourteen can look androgynous. Many male adolescents at these ages look quite soft and pretty. There is no beard, or consolidation of the child's facial features into an adult masculine configuration. With a superficial glance, one often does not know whether a young person of this age is male or female. The effeminate nature of the young adolescent male belongs to the "intersexual stage of the son-lover" (Neumann 1973, 157). Neumann saw this early stage of ego consciousness represented in the mythology of the son-lover's relationship to the Great Mother Goddess:

> Attis, Adonis, Tammuz, and Osiris figures in the Near Eastern cultures are not merely born of a mother. . . they are (also) their mother's lovers; they are loved, slain, buried, and bewailed by her, and are then reborn through her. The figure of the son-lover follows the stages of embryo and child. By differentiating himself from the unconscious and reaffirming his masculine otherness, he very nearly becomes the partner of the maternal unconscious. He is her lover as well as her son, but he is not yet strong enough to cope with her. He succumbs to her in death and is devoured. . . . The masculine principle is . . . still youthful and vernal, the merest beginning of an independent movement away from the place of origin and the infantile relation. . . . [These] flower-like boys are not sufficiently strong to resist and break the power of the Great Mother. They are more pets than lovers. (Neumann 1973, 47–8, 51)

Many adolescents become caught in this stage of early adolescence. Often, they become deeply involved with marijuana. One sixteen-year-old psychotic boy, heavily addicted to pot, told me his lady love was "Mary Jane," a colloquialism then current for marijuana. Such adolescents languish in a haze of "grass," unable to find motivation for anything.

> Case C: "C" could be called a true fertility god, proudly and carefully tending his field of marijuana cultivated in the woods near his home. He wore the plant symbol on his tee-shirt, home-made tattoo on his arm, and doodled it over and over when bored. He wore a big brass buckle with the pot insignia, given to him by his adoring mother, who could also scream at him in witch-like manner, (he reported), throwing him out to go live with his father (he would never stay long). His hair hung to his shoulders, covering a soft pretty face from which soulful eyes gazed, often rolled in exasperation at his mother.

Mothers can relate to their pubescent sons (between ages eleven and thirteen) with such intensity that there is an aura of sexual excitement between the two. In the privacy of a family therapy session, these boys' eyes stay riveted to their mother's faces.

Case A: "A's" mother reclined on the sofa during a family therapy session and placed her stocking feet in her young son's lap while his father just sat haplessly. Chuckling, she and her husband told how their "baby" (A) used to hit father in the shins when the latter returned from Vietnam eleven years earlier and dared to hug his wife. "A" did not seem uncomfortable with Mom's feet in his lap, nor with this story.

The transition from child to adolescent is also marked by the emergence of fear and a death feeling as the ego "steps forth from the magic circle . . . and finds itself in loneliness and discord" (Neumann 1973, 114). Sexual desire and orgasm is experienced as "all-powerful transpersonal phallus and womb. . . . The mother is still too great an influence and is transformed into the "Terrible Mother," who, as enchantress, confuses the senses and drives men out of their minds. No adolescent can withstand her. [D]issolution of personality and of individual consciousness [can result, for] insanity is an ever-recurring symptom of possession by her. . . ." (Neumann 1973, 61).

Case E: A thirteen-year-old blond, pudgy, moonfaced, pubescent boy practiced session after session shooting rubber-tipped darts at targets or building castles and staging battles between two armies of G. I. Joe and Zartan, the Chameleon Man. The battles were notable by their remarkable variety of guns and shooting escapades. The boy seemed to be trying to build up masculinity. His draw-an-opposite-person on a psychological test was an "evil-looking" female creature whose lower body ended in a pointed tail. When initially hospitalized (the previous year), he had clung to his mother with such force, wailing and crying, that he eventually had to be subdued by five members of the staff. The symbiotic tie between mother and son was almost physically visible. Now, the rush of sexual feelings and eruptions of hallucinatory rage had necessitated his being rehospitalized. He had attacked his mother and sister with a fireplace poker. He had also threatened his mother with a knife—to cut the cord? [3]

Strugglers

In Neumann's stage of the Twins or Strugglers, the young person has become aware of him/herself and begins to say, "No!" to the *uroboros*, to the Great Mother, to the pull of unconsciousness. As Neumann puts it, "[t]he motto of all consciousness is *determinatio est negatio* . . . I am not that!" (1973, 121). The Twin or Struggler feels divided because the acquisition of an ego does not do away with the formidable other side, which resists the process of becoming conscious. Doubt may drive him or her to desperation, suicide, murder of the ego, and a self-mutilation that culminates in death. The parental imagoes, especially the mother, are seen as instruments of dangerous, overwhelming oppression to be avoided or met with fear.

The young adolescent experiences part of the destructive force formerly belonging to the Terrible Mother as a personal possession. This destructive tendency is assimilated through self-mutilation, suicidal thoughts, and suicide attempts. The ego has begun to gain control over the aggressive tendency formerly projected onto the mother and/or father, and to make it a content of consciousness.

> Case F: A fourteen-year-old girl confided that she still was very afraid of her parents when they got angry. She also said that she felt excited and nonplussed about "accidentally" setting fire to nearby woods with firecrackers (M-80's) while her male friends looked scared. She seemed to enjoy the power of this destructive act. Earlier in the year, she had picked hairs out of her knuckles and forearms, and had cut on herself within the pubic hair line. She also insisted on piercing her ear lobes with an unsterilized pin a second time against the orders of her parents.

The insecurity produced by the sense of continuing division into opposing psychic systems (i.e., ego consciousness *vs.* unconsciousness) can also lead to profound doubt, which is manifested in narcissism and *Weltschmerz* (world sadness). Egocentricity and self-absorption, traits so characteristic of adolescence, are exaggerations of one's own importance and result from the adolescent's very recent emancipation from the unconscious. On the other hand, egocentricity is compensated by self-destructive *Weltschmerz* and unconscious self-hatred.

In Neumann's view, the phase of the strugglers has a legitimate place in puberty. The ego which thinks of killing itself is more active, more independent, and more individual than the sad resignation of the languishing son-lover. Neumann considered the self-destructive acts and tragic self-division of the struggler to be heroic.

Case B: "B" was a fourteen-year-old male who looked like a flower-child of the sixties, with flowing shoulder-length hair that covered half his face. There were scars from cigarette burns on his forearms from playing "chicken" by himself or with other boys. He had made three suicide attempts, but said the first two were accidental because he was "freaked out" on drugs and alcohol. He had also run away several times, placing himself in danger by hitchhiking. The third attempt at death involved taking every pill he could find in his mother's bathroom cabinet. He said he had just wanted to go to sleep and never wake up. He told me that going to the hospital, detention home, or otherwise being separated from his parents was a fate worse than death. The day he overdosed he had received a court sentence for assaulting a female teacher.

Case A: "A" had torn apart a hospital unit and had been transferred because he was incorrigible. His latest suicide attempt had been his most serious: a cocktail of medication, street drugs, and alcohol. He was filled with self-hatred when I first met him. His older brother had shot himself in the abdomen with a shotgun two years earlier and, miraculously, had lived. "A" felt no reason to live.

Case D: A fifteen-year-old girl, "D," repeatedly ran away from adoptive parents, hung around anti-social friends, got into minor scrapes with the law, and then earnestly and sincerely promised never to do such things again. On one runaway, she spent several bitterly cold nights under the house of an acquaintance. When she was lying and stealing, she was constantly thinking about suicide. At other times she was sweetly cooperative, academically and socially adept, and a born leader. This was the 'old "D"' that her parents used to know before she reached adolescence. In her therapy sessions, she was full of self-loathing, and expressed disbelief concerning her self-destructive behavior. She had an inexplicable longing to get pregnant, yet "knew better"; however she haphazardly exposed herself to the possibility of pregnancy. She was divided against herself at fundamental levels. Her situation was made more complicated by the fact that she had been adopted as a little girl. Not only was she divided against herself, but she was struggling with a mother imago that contained both a "bad" mother (natural mother in prison for writing bad checks, from whom she had been taken at age three because of abuse and neglect), and a "good" mother (adoptive mother who took her and her sister into a loving Christian family).

Case G: A fifteen-year-old girl stole the family car and engaged in a high speed chase with the police, crashing into a barrier erected to stop her. In the hospital, she introduced herself as Jennifer. Her given name was Pam. She said she "does bad things" when she is Pam, but is a popular cheerleader type when she is called Jennifer. She thought often of death and suicide. She engaged in promiscuous sex with boys in a pathetic, wild, party-girl manner. She struggled desperately with her sense of self-division by trying to fit in with her environment no matter the cost. She lied to please whomever she was with. Her dreams were full of grisly images from horror films in which mutilation, dismemberment, and death were paramount.

It is during the phase of the Strugglers or Twins that adolescents first become self-conscious.[4] Then, they feel the self-alienation and self-estrangement that are hallmarks of the essential doubleness of consciousness. These more severely disturbed adolescents manifest compelling themes of despair, destruction, love, hate, rebellion, clinging, and fear, themes that give us a window into the archetypal underpinnings of the adolescent psyche during this phase of development.

Trickster

In order to conform to reality, the ego's will to power must give way to laws of inner change or outer necessity. This submission does not come easily or automatically for the youth. During early adolescence, the Trickster-figure might be an archetypal source of the resistance to the change needed to acquire ego strength. The Trickster "knows no difference between right and wrong, accepts no discipline other than his own experimental attitudes toward life" (Henderson 1979, 36). Although not mentioned by Neumann, the Trickster would seem to be an intermediate stage between the Struggler and the Hero.

The Trickster is an archetypal figure whose physical appetites dominate his behavior.[5] He has the emotional mentality of an infant: low frustration tolerance and no ability to delay gratification. In addition, he is often cruel, cynical, unfeeling, and mischievous. In general, the Trickster is identifiable by a generally prominent phallic and/or magical attribute, a shape-changing ability, a proclivity for inflicting (and suffering) pain and injury, sly humor, impulsiveness, and meddlesome curiosity. One of the Trickster's outstanding characteristics is an abysmal lack of consciousness: "He does the most atrocious things from sheer unconsciousness and unrelatedness." (Jung 1954, 473).

Mythological tricksters include North American Coyote, alchemical Mercurius, Norse Loki, Chinese Monkey, Greek Prometheus, Hermes, Lucifer, the Italian Pulcinella, Merlin, Punch, Br'er Rabbit, Curious George, and Charlie Chaplin's Little Tramp. These figures' fondness for sly jokes and malicious pranks, their powers as shape-shifter, their dual nature (half-animal, half-divine), an exposure to all kinds of tortures, and an approximation to the figure of savior all indicate the presence of Trickster.

Case B: "B," the fourteen-year-old with flowing, shoulder-length curly hair and cigarette burns on his arms embodied many trickster features. Viewed from behind, he looked like a girl, especially in the way he walked; from the front, he was a tough boy-man with a sly mischievous grin. He was both an earnestly compliant, sweet child, and an angry snarling animal, who literally bared his teeth at his therapist. During the first session he cried in the forlorn manner of a waif; in the second session, he greeted the therapist with a belligerent, "Suck my dick!" Phallic and aggressive themes emerged again when, in an outburst of psychotic rage during a family therapy session, he jumped up and yelled, "I'll cut your head off, nail it to the wall and use your mouth for a urinal!" On his forearm was the tattoo, "Dr. B." "Dr. B." expressed both his wish to be a healer (he had had aspirations of becoming a doctor when he was younger), and his function as drug supplier to his friends.

When medication had made "B" more psychotic, he was transferred to a unit for psychotic youngsters with tighter structure and was taken off the medication. There, he began to respond to the extremely firm and consistent rules and caring of the staff. When his parents supplied external controls on a pass, he said later they had "passed the test this weekend." This clearly illustrated his need to be contained through firm, non-vindictive confrontation by adults. He began to emerge as a leader on his unit, taking on a hero's

> role. One day while he was walking on a path in the woods, a snake dropped before him, hanging at eye level from a tree. He knocked it to the ground, killed it under his boot heel, skinned it, and proudly took his trophy home to pin on the wall. Was this his dragon fight?
>
> His relationship with his adoring, peer-like mother became more distant. Conversely, he became closer to his boundary-setting father. His parents worked out so many standards and rules by the time of discharge that he called his house "Home Institute" after the hospital (Colonial Institute) that had helped him to sufficiently transform his trickster (and struggler) energy, enabling him to get on with his development.

MTV provides a wealth of tricksterism—fast cuts, outlandish situations, sly humor, winks, inflicting and receiving pain, instant gratification, violence, sex, outrageous and witless actions, phallic and magical phenomena. On the adolescent's favorite television channel, all the laws of gravity, good taste, fashion, tradition, and the art of movie-making and recording seem to be made in order to be broken. Lawlessness is the law. What maturity sees as lawlessness, however, adolescence views as creativity and vitality.[6] Trickster energy, often seen as noxious and/or nonsensical by the adult on-looker, may nevertheless be a developmental necessity for the adolescent.

The archetype of the Trickster seems to embody "a kind of divinely sanctioned lawlessness that promises to become heroic" (Henderson 1979, 36). In the Winnebago trickster cycle, Coyote gradually evolves from a brutal, savage, and stupid animal into a useful and sensible being with many human attributes. In "Breakfast Club," a movie about five adolescents, a young hoodlum gradually takes on more heroic and human qualities. He develops from a mindlessly destructive trickster to a tricky hero whose actions save the others. In the end, he is given a diamond (often a symbol of the Self) by one of the girls.

Hero

Mythology is replete with images depicting the contest between the hero and the power of evil, often personified as a dragon or some other monster. These ancient stories and fairy tales portray the struggle of primitive humankind to achieve consciousness. In the development of consciousness, the hero is the "means by which the emerging ego overcomes the inertia of the unconscious mind, and liberates the maturing person from regressive longings" (Henderson 1964, 118). "The hero's main feat is to overcome the monster of darkness: it is the long-hoped-for and expected triumph of consciousness over unconscious" (Jung 1934, 284). Whenever the ego needs strengthening, symbols of the hero arise. Not surprisingly, the hero myth has meaning for the adolescent who is trying to discover and assert his or her own personality. As Henderson (1964) put it, "the essential function of the hero's myth is the development of the individual's ego-consciousness—his awareness of his own strengths and weaknesses in a manner that will equip him for the arduous tasks with which life confronts him" (112).

Case A: "A" had been a true son-lover of his mother. He enacted the role of "sexy boy" on the unit, relating to all women, young and old, staff and patients, in a flagrantly seductive manner. Struggler and Trickster were both present. When he wasn't depressed, he was cocky and mischievous, often brash, and always dramatic and "full of himself." He drove all but the most experienced staff to distraction, even despair, as they tried to hold the line and meet his challenge. He seemed to be testing their mettle.

Then quietly and gradually another aspect began to show. He began to talk about his dreams, often sketching them as he described the action in them. A gentle, but firm teacher began to tame him. He wrote a fairy tale he called "Beauty and the Beast." He wrote songs to play on his guitar. He identified with a deep-thinking rock star/songwriter (Jim Morrison) whose biography he was reading. Morrison had committed suicide and "A" explored what suicide might mean. He talked about his brother's almost fatal suicide attempt and about the broader issues of life and death.

"A's" name was that of a Celtic hero. He listened with interest to his namesake's legend. Shortly after, he had the following dream:

It is a bare, freshly painted room, bright yellow with an open passageway and a deck on the second story of a building by the sea. It is a bright sunny day. It is very bright in the room. There are guns on the floor, rifles like deer rifles, maybe four or five in a row. I come into the room. I can't remember before, but know there were people in it. There are windows all along one wall looking out on a bright sunny scene, very light.

"A" exhibited an enormous amount of manic excitement and energy in telling this dream. The next night he organized a "barricade" on the hospital unit, blocking the hall with furniture and taking over a room with another boy and two girls. Furniture was piled high against the door. When told of the episode, I was reminded of the fierce IRA fighters struggling in Northern Ireland against British soldiers. The staff calmed "A" and his confederates; the next morning they came out of the room of their own accord. The room and furniture sustained damage, but no one was harmed, and neither girl became pregnant. They had been contained.

The dream had been full of the masculine principle (symbolized in the bright sunlight and the rifles). From an archetypal viewpoint, "A" had been infused with masculine energy. "A's" father, though a professional soldier, was a rather distant, passive figure in the boy's experience. Still, the father bore the quintessential heroic name of a legendary Celtic king. "A" had fought the First Parents in the guise of the unit staff and structure. He had "killed the dragon" in a symbolic, albeit concrete and enacted manner. Something significant had occurred within his psyche. "A" acted the hero after his escapade, swaggering a bit, but calmer and more self assured. Peers looked up to him as leader. The blatant, brash sexuality was modulated. He no longer felt depressed. Two weeks later, "A" dreamed about his maturing masculinity:

I was somewhere with this guy named "Ting" (from Thailand) who plays the guitar. A big concert was going to happen that night. I told him: "I want to play a Flying-V," a guitar I don't usually like. We went through the halls to the backstage rooms. He went back and set it down. Ting said "It has gold hardware." It was a white Stratocaster with gold hardware on it, the exact opposite of my black/silver guitar. I picked it up and went right front of stage. I plugged the guitar into my box and we started playing "A Whole Lot of Loving Going On." First my guitar wasn't loud enough and I turned it up and I really got off to it waving my guitar. There were two other guitar players and a drummer backing me.

Thus, in the dream, an oriental "twin" joins the dream ego and gives him a new guitar, one that is trimmed in gold. Ting may symbolize the spiritual friend from the East who brings the higher masculinity to "A." This new guitar is the exact opposite of "A's" own guitar which was trimmed in the feminine silver. Gold may symbolize masculinity. White is associated with light and consciousness, black with dark and unconsciousness. The dream ego takes the stage and stands on the right or conscious side. He begins to play his own music, gradually turning up the volume. He is turned "way up." He is backed by three other masculine figures to make a quaternity of masculine wholeness on stage.

"A" was released from the hospital within three months. One early morning, he appeared for his outpatient appointment clad only in shorts and tennis shoes. He seemed to want to show off his tanned, muscular, man's body. Indeed, he had been a soft, white and pudgy boy when he had been admitted to the hospital in late January. He grew several inches, and now he looked like a tan, strong young man. Six weeks before discharge in June, he had dreamt:

I am muscular, skinny and tan. I am looking down at my arms which are powerful. My hand is clenched in pumping iron fashion. I am looking at my veins and the baby oil spread on my skin.

He had begun to take hold. He came two more times and then was gone, out into the world, away from his parents' home.

The adolescent girl comes to her heroic dragon fight in a different manner. Whereas the young male has to fight his way out of the maternal *uroborus*, the girl must moderate and subdue her yearning for the safety of the familial circle in order to make her own way as a mature woman. Her mother is her own kind; she is not Other. In the pictures of St. George and the Dragon, we see the maiden standing quietly with the dragon on a leash. These paintings suggest that the girl must not fight the dragon, but rather she must tame it and stay related to it. Neumann wrote that "the feminine way of defeating the dragon is to accept it" (1976, 121).

It has been said the culture makes boys into men and nature makes girls into women, that a woman's "lower nature" effects more of the separation from home. The female adolescent passage seems to involve a descent through nature rather than an ascent through spirit. Boys have to be *made* men through initiatory practices, conducted by male elders, while girls' rites are based more on the natural events of becoming women through menarche and pregnancy, or *growing* into women.[7]

The myth of Demeter and Persephone provides archetypal underpinnings for the coming and going of daughters with mothers.[8] Demeter searches in great distress for her daughter Persephone when the latter is abducted by Hades, king of the underworld. During spring and summer they are reunited; Persephone then returns to Hades as his queen. Adolescent daughters come and go from their mothers; they are sometimes close, sometimes distant. In less troubled pairings, the mother lets the daughter go, often in small ways emotionally and psychologically, and gladly receives her back as the daughter gradually evolves into a woman conscious of herself, separate yet related. In symptomatic families, the daughter's separation can go awry: she runs away repeatedly, and the parents angrily search for her and bring her back.

> Case D: "D" ran away in a cyclical, compulsive manner. She seemed to prefer darker companions (black boyfriends) on these runaways. She was not solidly grounded in a good enough mother. Although her adoptive mother was sweet and nurturing, her natural mother (who had raised her until age three) had been abusive, neglectful, and was currently in prison. Only by being imprisoned on the adolescent unit or in a detention home could "D" stop running. She went from our psychiatric unit to a Baptist Children's Home, and then to the State Girls' Correctional Facility. Perhaps her identification was with the mother who was locked up.

These troubled girls require a therapeutic approach which helps them to re-establish a bond with their mothers or some other nurturing feminine figure. Once she and her mother discover that their bond is greater than the anger and hurt of (necessary) separation, the family is able to continue its life cycle with less disastrous disruptions. The mother is able to let the daughter come and go, and the daughter leaves and returns of her own accord in a gradually widening arc.

Initiate

The will to achieve ego consciousness is part of the heroic phase of adolescent development. Once ego consciousness has been attained, however, there "comes a time to give up scaling mountains to prove strength and submit to a meaningful ritual of initiatory change that could fit the youth for responsibilities of maturity" (Henderson 1964, 132). Although the ordeal or trial of strength in initiation, (Neumann's fourth phase within adolescence) seems similar to the hero's ordeals, there is a fundamental difference between the initiate and the hero. The hero exhausts his ambition, succeeds in his labors, and then may die or be sacrificed. In contrast, the initiate is called upon to give up all desire, ambition, and especially will; he or she must submit to the ordeal and most often lives. Moreover, the initiate must be willing to experience this trial without hope of success. Initiates must be prepared to die, but most often prevail and become adult members of their community.

Through symbolic death, the ordeal of initiation returns the novice to the original unity of mother-and-child (Henderson 1964). Ego identity, then, is dissolved in initiatory rites—often via some concrete form of dismemberment. The ordeal may be *mild*: tattooing, tooth knocked out, fasting; or, it may be *agonizing*: circumcision, sub-incision, mutilation, or lying in the hot sun for hours without moving a muscle. The purpose of this initiation is to rescue the neophyte from unity with the Mother and to bring about a rebirth of the ego within the adult group or collective, i.e., a totem, clan, or tribe. Thus, the adolescent male is initiated into the collective entity of heaven, father, and spirit. The tribal girl's rite of passage is centered on first menstrual cycle or on breast budding, whereby the adolescent female becomes a woman among women, participating fully in the collective life of her community as a marriageable female.

Contemporary adolescents enact these archetypal themes of initiation on their own (i.e.,without help from the adult collective). They may wear outrageous punk styles with bizarre haircuts (e.g., Mohawk, or one side of hair shaved) and colors. Multiple piercing of the earlobe is also very popular, as is tattooing. "B," for example, had tattooed "Dr. B" on his forearm; and "C" had earned money by tattooing his friends. More disturbed teenagers may mutilate themselves. Scarification is the result. Initiation hunger may also underlie many of today's teenage pregnancies.

Victor Turner (1977) called the second phase of the rite of passage a marginal or *liminal* period in which the state of the initiate or "passenger" is ambiguous. The most characteristic symbol of this liminal state is that of paradox, of being both this and that, of being living and dead, of being *androgynous*. The world of music is replete with such ambiguous images, with androgyny becoming ascendant in the 1980's. Michael Jackson, for example, has been described as "a chameleon-like being who is everything at once: male and female, black and white, violent and sweet, ascetic and gaudy. Nothing is surrendered; he has mingled all the opposites" (Rubenstein, 1984, 70). Along with Michael Jackson, Boy George and Prince, "set a new standard in androgynous allure" (Griffin 1984, 100). Mick Jagger and David Bowie were earlier examples of the androgynous appeal of rock stars. Similarly, Annie Lennox used to dress like "Elvis in Fifties drag" in music videos. Today, as she dresses in doubled breasted pantsuits and slicks back her short hair, k.d. lang looks like a handsome young man.

A formerly hospitalized psychotic adolescent wrote to me just before her eighteenth birthday. She clearly described initiatory themes of ordeal, death, and rebirth:

> I've been having trouble sleeping at night with nightmares. It's not really a dream, it's more of a hallucination. Seems like I die every night. . . . I lay down on my bed and then I feel like I bloat up real big. Then it feels like I am floating. Then my breathing gets real shallow. I go with it scared I am already dead. . . . I stay awake too scared to sleep. My x-spirits . . . say if I make it I will die to some extent. I have a vision of dying and my old spirit getting up and leaving my body. I wake up and am a totally new woman. . . . I see myself as having a very successful future. If I make it.

The Waning of Projected Archetypes

During childhood, children project the archetype of the First Parents onto their parents and the parents project the archetype of the Child onto their child. Adolescence, however, is different. It is a time of declining parental archetypal activity. In adolescence, the child must come to terms with his parents as real people, accepting their deficiencies as well as their strengths. Similarly, the parents must be ready to give up their archetypal identification with the First Parents and to withdraw their projections of Child from their teenager.

There are four possible outcomes: 1) the child withdraws projections from the parents, but the parents do not withdraw their Child projections from the adolescent; 2) parents withdraw their projections, but the adolescent does not; 3) both sides withdraw their projections more or less simultaneously; and 4) both sides persist and do not withdraw their projections (Stevens 1983).

Outcomes One and Two are one-sided and quite problematic. A child who withdraws the projection of First Parent will become rebellious if the parents refuse to withdraw their projection of Child. Conversely, if the parents prematurely withdraw their projection of Child before their teenager is ready, then the teenager may be pushed into clinging and anxious attachment. If this situation becomes chronic, the teenager may become mired in a lifelong pursuit of parent-substitutes.

Outcome Three, that is, the timely mutual withdrawal of projections, is the healthy developmental course. Outcome Four, on the other hand, is disastrous for both as the young person and parents remain bound together and the emerging young adult is prevented from taking his or her appropriate place in the adult collective.

Psychic Inertia and Fear of the New

Two factors make it difficult for adolescents to separate from their childhood home: psychic inertia and avoidance of the new. Psychic inertia manifests itself as resistance to change, but is essential for a sense of permanence and stability in consciousness:

> We experience psychic inertia most powerfully where parental archetypes are involved. Attempts to run counter to the established childhood patterns can strike the [adolescent as well as] the adult with terror because these patterns have been incorporated under the spell of what every child experiences as the parents' magical or god-like authority (Whitmont 1978, 124–5).

Our sense of security is so tied to the familiar that change may be felt as a threat of death, or extinction. Such threat may be maximized when change of status is being negotiated within the archetypal parental haze. The struggle takes on the illusion of life and death magnitude. Then, Outcome One may lead to rebellious thoughts of murder. Outcome Two may result in anxiety and fear of dying. Even the healthy Outcome Three must cause sadness and mourning as the old order passes away.

Avoidance of the new is first seen in the stranger anxiety of the eight-month-old infant who clings to mother. In adolescence, the teenager is struggling with the greatest change of his or her life. As a result, teenagers may need help in moving forward. Rites of initiation can help to overcome psychic inertia and fear of the new by "providing the symbols and the group impetus needed to carry the libido forward and to loosen the ties holding it back" (Stevens 1983, 147).

Therapists must keep in mind such inertia and fear as they deal with teens and their families. Therapy, both individual and family, can provide the initiation process that today's society so rarely provides for its young people. The adolescent is a liminar in today's culture, occupying the interstices and margins of society, being neither this nor that, the quintessential paradoxical being. His and her "monstrous" enactments can broaden our own definition of what it is to be human. But we, (as therapists and parents), must meet the challenge if the children of our society are to successfully join the community as responsible adults.

Notes

1. The English word *adolescence* can be traced back to Middle English, spoken after the Norman invasion of 1066, between 1100 and 1500 A.D. The word has its origins in the Latin and French *alere*, to nourish and *alescere*, to begin to grow. Joining *ad* to the latter gives us *adolescere*, connoting "to grow up."

2. Infant observation research since Neumann's writing has contributed empirical data to augment and modify Neumann's more intuitive perspective. For instance, the infant may have the illusion of oneness with the mother in the first few months of life, but is considered a unique separate being from *in utero* (see Stern 1985; Piontelli 1987, 453; Miller 1989; Sidoli 1989; Piontelli 1992).

3. Neumann stated that sexuality perceived as losing ego-consciousness and feeling overpowered by the female was an archetypal experience in puberty for males (1973, 60–1).

4. I would like to develop examples using females for all of Neumann's classifications in another paper. The Strugglers phase easily included girls.

5. There are few examples of female tricksters in the literature. One that comes to mind is Agnes Whistling Elk, a shaman depicted in Lynn Andrews' book. In a recent book,*Mercury Rising: Women, Evil, and the*

Trickster Gods, my colleague, Deldon A. McNeely, presents her explorations of the feminine Trickster.

6. "So to see ourselves, we turn our eyes where our parents turn up their noses—MTV. With its glitzy, jumpy, sound- and video-bite format, its semi-multicultural flavor, MTV celebrates our creativity and vitality, and validates the confusion of growing up in an era of ambiguity" (Jones 1994, B7).
7. An account of a puberty ritual among the women of the Cuna tribe in Panama is eloquently presented in "Mu Olokukurtilisop" (Stone 1984, 78–9). Painting the face with red juice may also be found among the menarche rituals of the Navajo.
8. From a private conversation with my colleague, Ron Schenk, who had lived and worked on reservations in New Mexico, I have learned that there is also a ritual custom during puberty ceremonies among the Navajo of a girl's running away into the desert and her return.

References

Andrews, L. 1982. *Medicine Woman.* San Francisco: Harper & Row.

Campbell, J. 1973. *Hero with a Thousand Faces.* Bollingen Series 17. Princeton, N. J.: Princeton University Press.

Campbell, J., and B. D. Moyers. 1988. Videocassette. The hero's adventure.*The Power of Myth.* Program One. New York: Mystic Fire Video, Inc.

Davis, M., and Wallbridge, D. 1981. *Boundary and Space: An Introduction to the Work of D. W. Winnicott.* New York: Brunner/Mazel.

Erikson, E. H. 1968. *Identity, Youth and Crisis.* New York: W.W. Norton & Co.

Fordham, M., Gordon, R., Hubback, J., and Lambert, K., eds. 1985. *Explorations into the Self.* London: Academic Press.

Fordham, M. 1976. *The Self and Autism.* Library of Analytical Psychology. Vol. 3. London: William Heinemann Medical Books, Ltd.

Griffin, N. 1984. The most. *Life*, September, 87–100.

Henderson, J. 1964. Ancient myths and modern man. In *Man and His Symbols.* Ed. C. G. Jung. New York: Doubleday & Co., Inc.

______. 1979. *Thresholds of Initiation.* Middletown, Conn.: Wesleyan University Press.

Jones, A. N. 1994. Newspapers took youth seriously after Cobain died. *Virginian Pilot and Ledger Star.* B7.

Jung, C. G. 1902. Psychology of so-called occult phenomena. In *CW* 1: 3–88. Princeton, N. J.: Princeton University Press, 1975.

———. 1931. The stages of life. In *CW* 8: 387–403. Princeton, N. J.: Princeton University Press, 1978.

———. 1934. The relations between the ego and the unconscious. In *CW* 7: 123–72. Princeton, N. J.: Princeton University Press, 1977.

———. 1946. Psychic conflicts in a child. In *CW* 17: 1–36. Princeton, N. J.: Princeton University Press, 1977.

———. 1954. On the psychology of the trickster-figure. In *CW* 9: 255–74. Princeton, N. J.: Princeton University Press, 1977.

Kaplan, L. J. 1984. *Adolescence: The Farewell to Childhood.* New York: Simon & Schuster.

McNeely, Deldon. 1996. *Mercury Rising: Women, Evil, and the Trickster Gods.* Dallas: Spring.

Miller, L., Rustin, M., and Shuttleworth, J., eds. 1989. *Closely Observed Infants.* London: Gerald Duckworth & Co., Ltd.

Neumann, E. 1973. *The Origins and History of Consciousness.* Tr. R. F. C. Hull. Princeton, N. J.: Princeton University Press.

———. 1976. *The Child.* Tr. Ralph Manheim. New York: Harper Colophon.

Piontelli, A. 1987. Infant observation from before birth. *International Journal of Psychoanalysis* 68 (1987): 453–63.

———. 1992. *From Fetus to Child: An Observational and Psychoanalytic Study.* New York: Routledge.

Rubenstein, C. 1984. The Michael Jackson syndrome. *Discover: The Newsmagazine of Science,* September: 69–70.

Sidoli, M. 1989. *The Unfolding Self: Separation and Individuation.* Boston: Sigo Press.

———, and Davies, M., eds. 1988. *Jungian Child Psychotherapy Individuation in Childhood.* London: Karnac Books.

Stern, D. N. 1985. *The Interpersonal World of the Infant: A View from Psychoanalysis and Developmental Psychology.* New York: Basic Books.

Stevens, A. 1983. *Archetypes: A Natural History of the Self.* New York: Quill.

Turner, V. 1969. *The Ritual Process: Structure and Anti-Structure.* Chicago: Aldine Publishing Co.

_____. 1973. *Dramas, Fields and Metaphors.* Ithaca: Cornell University Press.

_____. 1977a. Process, system and symbol: new anthropological synthesis. *Daedalus* 106.3 (Summer): 61–75.

_____. 1977b. Variations on a theme of liminality. In *Secular Ritual.* Ed. S. Moore and B. Meyerhoff. Amsterdam: Van Gorcum & Co.

_____. 1982. *From Ritual to Theatre.* New York: Performing Arts Journal Publications.

Van Gennep, A. 1908. 1960. *The Rites of Passage.* Tr. M. B. Vizedom and G. L. Caffee. Chicago: University of Chicago Press.

Whitmont, E. C. 1978. *The Symbolic Quest.* Princeton, N. J.: Princeton University Press.

Wickes, F. 1927. 1966. *The Inner World of Childhood.* Englewood Cliffs, N. J.: Prentice-Hall, Inc.

Winnicott, D. W. 1965. Adolescence: struggling through the doldrums. In*The Family and Individual Development.* London: Tavistock.

_____. 1982. *Playing and Reality.* London: Tavistock.

Sue Crommelin, *L.C.S.W., is a Diplomat in Jungian Psychology, and has over thirty years of experience in working with adolescents—as a youth group leader, mother, therapist, and analyst. She has taught Jungian psychology and family therapy at various conferences and meetings across the country, and in Norfolk, Virginia, where she now practices. Currently, Sue is using archetypal images of adolescence from modern American film, to demonstrate how archetypes play in the contemporary American imagination.*

Reclaiming Dream Lovers: Couples in Dialogue

Polly Young-Eisendrath

Introduction

Couple relationship begins early—before birth. The dependence that we have and feel for another person is our lifelong fate. There is no self except in relationship with another, and the repercussions from our earliest couple relationship extend throughout life. Early patterns of attachment, and the images or representations that accompany them, extend into lifelong habits of thought and action. Carl Jung called these habits "psychological complexes" and saw them as the central units of organization in the human personality (1969). Psychological complexes are experienced in adulthood as sub-personalities, as trance states—the associated mix of thoughts, images, sensations and impulses that cohere around an emotional core. When in a complex, we are "beside ourselves" in a familiar, but still alien way.

Human emotions universally compel us to organize our experiences into "good" and "bad," or "pleasant" and "irritating." Our actual human relationships in early life are carried forth later as styles or patterns of attachment. These styles of attachment are what psychoanalyst and researcher John Bowlby (1988), and his followers, have called "working models" that underlie secure, resistant or avoidant relational patterns.

Not only do we forever bring with us traces of our earliest couple relationships, but we organize a sense of identity as a *self* versus *other*, beginning with self-recognition at about eighteen months. This "identity couple" (self and other) develops as we develop. Eventually, the important other is the opposite sex, but initially our curiosity is directed to the parental others. When we are toddlers and young children, the question, "Who are They?" is typically addressed to our parents. Once upon a time, there was a King and a Queen . . . is the story of the parents' early power. Later "Who are They?" is directed to our same-sexed peers, and only later, especially in adolescence, does this whole drama usually shift to one permanently puzzling other—the opposite sex. "Who are They?"—as a question about the opposite sex—occupies many of us for a lifetime. We engage in a world that casts the two sexes mostly as antagonists (with the exception of romance, a brief period of idealizing projections); assigns them different power, status, and privilege; and also claims that it is "only natural" that they should pair up together in lifetime bonds. These conditions combine to create the opposite sex as a powerful projection-making factor, the "Other within" who carries fears, ideals, and wishes that we want to exclude from the self. (I capitalize Other to indicate that I am referring to a subjective state, a fantasized Other, and not to an actual person.)

The adult couple, then, carries all of the tendencies of both partners to see, feel, and understand each other as Parent and as outsider of the opposite sex, as a target for projection. Much of the remainder of this paper looks at the complexity of gender, envy, and power differences for adult heterosexual couples in patriarchy. The last section presents some specific steps that are characteristic of a couple in therapy who are successful in vitalizing their relationship. Although I work with same-sex couples using the therapeutic methods I will describe here, I am directing my comments primarily to heterosexual couples, especially because of the differences in power and meaning between the sexes. Many of my ideas apply also to same-sex couples, but the sameness of their gender identity creates a different fabric of relationship.

In this paper, I want to demystify heterosexual intimacy; heterosexuality has tended to be seen as something "natural." *Intimacy* between the sexes is anything but natural. It is achieved only through concentrated self-awareness, especially in regard to gender differences. In order to be intimate, partners must be friends. Long-term intimate friendship between the sexes, especially in marriage, is only now barely imaginable. Friendship is based on equality and mutuality, a condition that has not been possible for men and women until recently, as women have become speakers for themselves.

Acknowledging the complexity of male-female relationships, we can recognize the importance of *dialogue* as a means for establishing trust or empathy with the other sex. Dialogue is a special form of conversation that is grounded in different perspectives and a foundation of *trust* between participants. Only a foundation of trust will allow real differences to emerge. To have a dialogue, we must have two people who can speak *and* listen. Each must be *interested* in understanding the other, not simply in making a point. Both must be able to share in the horizon of meaning between them that develops from airing their respective points of view. In dialogue, we expect surprise and discovery. We assume that exchange will lead to an outcome previously unknown or unconscious for one or both participants. From all that I said earlier, you can probably imagine that dialogue is difficult for heterosexual couples.

After the romance has ended, when partners tend to comply with each other's needs, a committed couple is at risk of repeating patterns of child-parent complexes. In the second stage of a relationship—what I have dubbed "disillusionment"—couples enter into power struggles. During disillusionment, partners use active and passive aggression to deal with conflicts. They maintain systems of projection and projective identification in which both people are re-enacting dominance-submission patterns of early family relationships. Many couples do not resolve disillusionment. They adapt to it. Our culture (and other patriarchal cultures) supports the story of the "battle of the sexes," and fuels images of antagonism.

Many of our parents lived within the contract of marriage without intimate partnership. They were not best friends even if they did find ways to avoid open hostilities. They lived in perpetual fluctuations of hurt, resentment, despair, shame, and rage. Under these conditions, conversations take deadly forms. They may be paired monologues in which each partner holds forth in a solo speech. Or they may be repetitive exchanges that follow a predictable course of embattled positions. Neither person feels satisfied with the exchange and both find it boring because it is so predictable. Open attacks and fights often have the format of repetitive exchange. When disillusioned couples come for therapy, they have generally given up trying to talk things out. Usually both partners come with the goal that therapy should change the other, not the self.

Dialogue Therapy

As a feminist, Jungian psychoanalyst, developmental psychologist, and psychotherapist, I am dedicated to developing intimacy through dialogue. I am convinced that the eye-to-eye dyadic stance, the self in reflection, is the basis for psychological development throughout the lifespan. *Mirroring transformations* is my term for the reflections offered, and the boundaries clarified, of the self in intimate relationship. When a trusted partner (in marriage, friendship, or psychotherapy) offers a view, a criticism, or a compliment, the gesture carries heartfelt meaning that helps us transcend the limits of ourselves. The emphasis here is on *trust* because the discovery of new meaning that may promote development requires a basis of trust.

Together with my husband, Ed Epstein, I use a method of couple therapy that we originated and developed. We first called it "dyadic-dialogical therapy," but recently shortened that to Dialogue Therapy. This method is presented in detail in a book I published in 1984, *Hags and Heroes: A Feminist Approach to Jungian Psychotherapy with Couples*. The development of trust through dialogue therapy, and all that I have experienced in ten years of using it with many couples, is presented in a book I published in 1993, *You're Not What I Expected: Learning to Love the Opposite Sex*. This paper will summarize some central points from the second book, emphasizing especially the problem of projection and projective identification in couples.

Dialogue therapy is a method designed to work intensively and quickly (six sessions, one per month over six months, and a seventh session as a follow-up six months later). My husband and I (or other co-therapists who use the method) work as a dyadic team in emotionally intense encounters with couples. Each session is two hours long, during which the couple, facing each other, are directed into conversation while we, the therapists, sit slightly behind and out of the view of each partner. I sit behind the right shoulder of the woman, and my husband behind the left shoulder of the man. We are out of their fields of vision but fully attentive to what is going on. While the couple attempt to talk together, we act as "doubles" or "alter egos," and speak from the feelings and meanings that are implied but not claimed in what is being said. I try to empathize with the felt predicament of the woman, and my husband with the man. This method is designed to teach and encourage dialogue.

Partners learn how to maintain separateness (of their own thoughts and feelings) and openness (to listen with curiosity and interest). In this way, they come to claim and understand what has been excluded from the self as Other, and to disclaim and understand what is projected by the other partner. By disclaim, I mean that they learn to refuse to identify with, and/or be labeled as the single cause of fears, ideals, wishes, and unconscious fantasies of the partner. Increasingly, the partners gain a fundamental acceptance of their own subjective states. With this comes renewed vitality in the relationship. Partners come to feel confident about being able to talk about their differences without becoming entrapped in projective identification, the playing out of early dominance-submission routines with parents.

At this point, partners reach the goal of Dialogue Therapy—something I call "mature dependence," borrowing the term from psychoanalyst W. R. Fairbairn (1952). Mature dependence is the ability to give and take in a reciprocal manner. It requires being both dependent and dependable in a conscious way. Dependence is healthy and necessary for human beings over their lifespans, but it must change and develop from early clinging dependence to later mature dependence, an exchange of strengths.

Gender, Dream Lovers and Envy

To be a member of the human community is to be marked by a sign of "opposites" (female/male) and a requirement to join one of two exclusive clubs. These two clubs are created on the principle of division, the division of the world into two sexes and the requirements of gender applicable to each. This division into two groups creates an intrapsychic division as well—between the identity known as self and that known as Other. In each one of us live both personalities, one of a familiar gendered self, and another of a "strange gender," the excluded opposite. Both are emotionally charged with psychological complexes that arise and are sustained in a matrix of relationships. The division of the human community into two genders is both the separation of gendered persons into two groups, and the intrapsychic separation of the "I" from a "not-I" of the opposite gender.

Our strange gender is a powerful emotional determinant of development because of its unique relationship with the self. Strange gender constrains and limits the self. The way I act and imagine myself as a woman carries with it a tandem meaning of what I imagine to be male and masculine, what I see as human but "not-woman." These images, thoughts, impulses, and sensations cohere into a sub-personality of a masculine Other that is paradoxically the product of a female psyche. The same is true for the feminine Other in the male psyche.

Before I go further in detailing these multiple subjectivities, let me clarify the way I use the terms *sex* and *gender,* and how envy plays a role in casting the dream lovers of our strange gender. The "sex" we are born as and the "gender" we are assigned at birth (or even before birth now) are not the same thing, although one flows from the other. Sex is the difference of embodiment, the structural and functional properties of the human body, which includes both possibilities and constraints on who we can be. Sex is definite and inflexible in most cases. It provides for certain biological possibilities in male and female bodies. Breasts, vagina, vulva, womb, smaller body size, menstruation, pregnancy, lactation, menopause, and greater longevity are expected of a female body. Penis, greater body size, greater physical strength, impregnation, and lesser longevity are expected of the male body. These and other biological differences (e.g., the structure of the brain and hormonal chemistry) limit us in our biological-sexual-reproductive possibilities. Although we may struggle against these limitations (e.g., dressing as the other sex or attempting surgically to change the body) we cannot escape our sexual embodiment. It will limit us forever.

Gender, on the other hand, is more flexible. Gender consists of the characteristics, social roles, personality traits, power, and status that are assigned by society to each sex. Gender serves many purposes in the way societies organize work and power so that the tasks of life can get done. Gender varies by *context*—group, family, society. In some societies, for example, men are expected to be more nurturing and home-oriented than women, taking care of the young. In others, like our North American societies, women are expected to be the primary caregivers.

In my view, only *two* gender characteristics can be considered universal or nearly so. First, gender is a division into two groups that are exclusive. Second, women have less power than men in all male-dominated societies (i.e., most societies of the world). By less power, I mean that the work women do and the characteristics that are socially sanctioned for them tend to carry fewer privileges, smaller rewards, and reduced decision-making in comparison with those of men. These two characteristics of gender-dichotomy and unequal power, produce gender conflicts for women and men in relationship.

The biological differences of sex, and the dichotomy and power differences of gender, universally arouse troubling emotions about the opposite sex. Envy, jealousy, idealization and fear are the most common barriers to interpersonal trust. Intrapsychic barriers form around these emotions in both women and men, barriers that lead to psychological complexes of the opposite sex. I will talk more about these below.

First, I want to address the most confusing of these troubling emotions—envy. Both sexes envy the biological resources of the other. Using psychoanalyst Melanie Klein's (1975) definition, envy is a form of hatred that expresses the desire to *destroy* what another possesses because one cannot possess it for oneself. Envy is expressed as an attack that diminishes, empties, or belittles another. Envy is felt as emptiness in the self—a lack of resources that another possesses. In the felt emptiness, the only way to "even the score" is to destroy the worth, meaning, resources, or body of the other.

Each sex looks at the other's biologically ordained possibilities with the knowledge that these cannot be possessed by the self. Biological envy cannot be reduced to certain organs such as penis, breast, or womb because it is a shifting drama, based on limitations (e.g., in the chronicity of midlife illnesses, women see doctors six times more often than men and envy men's apparent health, but then men envy women's longevity in the average eight-year longer lifespan of women). Each sex has desires to belittle, destroy, dominate, or triumph over the other's biological possibilities and resources.

What about envy of gender differences? Isn't it a simple matter of women envying men? It is certainly true that female people envy the greater privileges and freedoms afforded to male people, characterized by psychoanalyst Nancy Chodorow (1978) as "phallus envy." It is also true, though, that male people envy the lesser privileges (and what is imagined to be fewer responsibilities) connected with being female. We North Americans are now in the peculiar situation of witnessing gender-based men's movement(s) that have evolved somehow in response to the women's movement(s). Many men seem to envy the clear and competent identities and emotional support and closeness that women have found among themselves in their searches for something better. Sometimes it seems as though some men envy the oppression that has mobilized and affected women.

Envy of the biological possibilities and gendered differences of the opposite sex limits our ability to see ourselves clearly *and* to empathize with others. Jung's (1959) original concepts of *anima* and *animus*, as opposite sex personalities arising from biological determinants in each sex, have been useful for me in coming to understand the function of envy. I have transformed these two terms into the projection-making complexes of "dream lovers"—those opposite sex Others who emerge full-blown from our socialization into a gendered self. Although I see dream lovers as products of culture and socialization, I believe they are critically important to our development in adulthood. Because of the enormous power of the gender dichotomy and the power differentials of the two sexes, our dream lovers unconsciously compel us to see ourselves and the opposite sex in certain ways that prevent full adult development if they remain unconscious.

By the time we reach adulthood, we have formed and defended a strong case of the strange gender. Our strange gender, the way we imagine the opposite sex, becomes emotionally powerful after we know that we cannot escape the singularity of our own gender and sex. At around the age of six or seven, children master the idea of gender exclusivity. At this point, fantasies and fears mix with envy as we turn to our same-sex peers to find out about ourselves *and* the opposite sex. Cultural stereotypes, media images, and all of the implied meanings conveyed by family and friends mix with our parental complexes to make dream lovers, those powerful Others who prowl through our night dreams and catch us unawares during the day.

Dream lovers begin as emotion-based images. They begin with the emotional forces that shape our ability to love and trust, even before they are associated in any way with the same or opposite sex. In our early years of greatest helplessness, parents and siblings or other caregivers engage us through care. Their voices, their faces, their ability (or inability) to be tender and available will mark us forever. *Emotional image traces* from early life collect around our needs and how they are met. These emotional traces gradually develop into psychological complexes, organized by core states of emotional arousal. Every complex is grounded in a particular set of images and meanings marked by emotion. For example, most of us have a "great mother complex" that is known to us through comfort and ease of sustenance and nurture, connected with sounds, smells, voice, and the handling of a woman. Initially we did not know of "woman" but later, when we understood the category, we assigned the term and perceived Mother as a woman. The early emotional image traces of a complex are not rational; they fall outside of language. The image traces orginated in actual experiences but those experiences were mostly nonverbal. They are hard to reach and understand later in life when they have infused our dream lovers with meanings that seem to "stem from the gut." They escape our ability to explain them. "I just *know* that you *hate* me because I can feel it in my body" can be so convincing to the person who feels the emotions, and yet so wrong about a partner.

As adults, our dream lovers can come between us and our best efforts to be fair with a spouse or friend of the opposite sex. It is not that dream lovers are specifically negative images of the opposite sex—not at all. Often they are idealized and inflated beliefs in the magical powers of the others. Dream lovers are simply "wrong" categories for understanding the actual others because they are rooted in our own subjectivity, sex, and gender. Dream lovers are felt through oneself, not through the other. They are assumptions that come under the sway of "I already *know*" what you are thinking or feeling, and so I don't need to ask.

Dream lovers are reinforced by our same-sex friends of childhood, adolescence, and adulthood. Dream lovers are fueled by stereotypes of "us" and "them," but they are rooted in psychological complexes. Challenging a complex, in oneself or another, is especially difficult because of the emotional core. The core is made of emotional image traces that are linked to survival (for example, aggression, joy, fear), and universal patterns of relationship. Certain relational themes (domination, attachment, submission) are universally connected to emotions spontaneously expressed in images the world over. Images of the Great Mother and the Great Father arise among all peoples and were considered by Jung to be evidence of an innate organization of human expression. He called these image-themes *archetypes*, meaning primary imprints. In Jung's last theory (1944–1961), archetypes are not mysterious forms that lie outside experience. They are not Platonic ideals or aspects of a fuzzy collective unconscious. They are universal human experiences of emotionally powerful images that predispose us to certain actions in a relational context. When your spouse gives you the "critical eye" while you are taking care of a task, you may feel this as a judgmental Terrible Parent, overwhelming and suffocating you with demands. You collapse into a sort of trance state and feel like a Victim Child who is vulnerable to abuse. You are trapped by a negative dream lover arising from within, but you believe your spouse has done it to you, through a simple glance.

In the romance stage of a heterosexual relationship we tend to project ideal dream lovers: Maiden Lover or Hero, Great Mother or Great Father. In disillusionment, we shift into negatively charged projections of Terrible Mother or Terrible Father. In the way I see these complexes, each dream lover has both a "self" and an "other" pole. When a woman projects her Hero, for example, and her male partner falls short of the standards, she often shifts into seeing him as a Lost Child, the original self pole of the complex. So the Hero dream lover involves *both* the qualities of her Hero (the man a woman would be) and the qualities of her Lost Child (someone who needs a Hero to lead her). Either pole of the dream lover can be activated. In my recent book (1993), I describe four common dream lovers in women, and four in men. By name, the strangers in women are the Terrible Father, the Great Father, the Hero, and the Underground Genius (dark erotic and creative man). The strangers in men are the Terrible Mother, the Great Mother, the Mistress Lover (Whore), and the Maiden Lover (Amazon, Madonna, Ingenue). These dream lovers are well known in our culture and are the subject of a lot of dramas and tales. Each of these dream lovers is rooted in the emotional image traces of psychological complexes, fueled by fantasies of the opposite sex, the not-me. As people learn to claim their own strange gender, they come to know aspects of themselves that were previously hidden, as well as talents and capacities that have been disclaimed. Reclaiming dream lovers is a major step in development in adult life, and often leads to more flexible gender boundaries and greater empathy for the opposite sex.

Mature Dependence through Dialogue

To engage the often painful process of reclaiming dream lovers, partners must be suffering from disillusionment, loss, or betrayal. Within the framework of commitment to their relationship—confronting barriers to intimacy—partners begin the process of recognizing dream lovers and establishing mature dependence. For heterosexual people especially, the challenge is great because of the ongoing gender stereotypes and inequities between the sexes. Reclaiming dream lovers means an end to blaming and making attacks on oneself or another through envy or idealization of the strange gender. It means asking questions and being interested in a partner's experience, rather than silencing or trivializing. Most of all, reclaiming dream lovers means coming to terms with the abuse, rejection, ideals, hopes, wishes, and potential that one has hidden from oneself, and projected onto the partner.

Working in dialogue therapy with many couples over time, I

have mapped out five major steps that are characteristic of couples who succeed in transforming disillusionment into mature dependence. Simply stated, the five steps are:

1. Recognizing the vulnerability of the self and accepting an attachment relationship as the ground of self;
2. Reclaiming one's own dream lovers;
3. Learning how to relate and function through dialogue, especially in areas of conflict and difference;
4. Claiming (not shirking) one's ability to engage in dialogue about all sorts of things, so that partners feel the common ground that provides basic trust;
5. Expanding the uses of dialogue into daily activities with others that encourage greater empathy, concern, and interest.

The core step in developing mature dependence is reclaiming dream lovers. This process often takes place in the first four sessions of dialogue therapy, and it depends on a lot of factors that are learned by couples in terms of their communications about conflict, and their ability to be empathic and differentiated. I have broken the process down into seven parts that will, I hope, flesh out the struggle that I have witnessed in most cases. Here is the way the process of reclaiming usually unfolds:

- Seeing how early attachment patterns carry over to current relating;
- Discovering one's major dream lovers, by examining the fears, ideals, and wishes one feels for one's partner;
- Knowing how one's dream lovers fit with parents' lived and unlived lives, hopes, and dreams;
- Taking responsibility for one's subjective states, dream lovers, and other complexes;
- Claiming one's desires, ideals, wishes, fears, aggression, jealousy, and envy by actively changing to make them one's own;
- Acknowledging the hurts one has caused in the past by projecting all of the above onto one's partner or others;
- Putting into action one's strange gender in some way that keeps it a conscious part of oneself.

In my view, the central goal of heterosexual intimacy is freeing the relational self to develop mature dependence. To me, this is what Jung meant in suggesting, as he did in a 1925 essay, that marriage could be a "psychological relationship." The state of mature dependence includes differentiation as an individual and empathy for one's partner. With the reclaiming of dream lovers, partners not only feel safer and more trusting in regard to handling differences, they also become generally more alert to the deep structures of gender and the damage caused by inequality between the sexes. Both partners—no matter their political leanings—have a remarkable awakening. They become convinced, as all good friends do, that equality is the basis of trust, even between the sexes.

Concluding Remarks

Sexual equality, like racial equality, is a lofty goal, not because it is wholly beyond us, in our ability to imagine such a world, but because it would mean a radical change in our whole way of life. If at this moment, for instance, women all over the world were suddenly compensated with equal pay for the work they do (at home and in the marketplace), all major economic systems would collapse. That is because these systems are founded on unpaid and underpaid labor performed largely by women. Yet, I have come to believe that we will live in sexual equality within the next hundred years. How can I believe this?

In the past, only the exceptional few—the sages or the poets or the mystics—were able to invest themselves in developing self-awareness. Now this possibility is available to masses of people, to those people who are groping for meaning outside of clear traditions and rules. Many of these people are engaged in couple relationships. Many of these relationships are caught in disillusionment. That is not new. What is new, and what is quite startling, sitting here at the end of the twentieth century, is that women and men are seeking equal partnership as part of marriage. The search for heterosexual partnership pushes us past the barriers of a self-protective view of gender, and a projective view of the opposite sex. The search for heterosexual partnership provides an opening to our unconscious strange gender, and to a self-awareness that returns the opposite to the self. This search is analogous to the search for extraterrestial intelligence, I think: we know it's out there, but are just now getting the tools to contact it.

References

Bowlby, J. 1988. *A Secure Base: Parent-Child Attachment and Healthy Human Development.* New York: Basic.

Chodorow, N. 1978. *The Reproduction of Mothering: Psychoanalysis and the Sociology of Gender.* Berkeley: University of California Press.

Fairbairn, W. R. 1952. *Psychoanalytic Studies of the Personality.* Boston: Routledge & Kegan Paul.

Jung, C. G. 1959. Aion. *CW* 9ii. 2nd ed. Princeton, N. J.: Princeton University Press.

———. 1969. *The Structure and Dynamics of the Psyche. CW* 11. 2nd ed. Princeton, N. J.: Princeton University Press.

Klein, M. 1975. *Envy and Gratitude & Other Works.* New York: Delacorte.

Young-Eisendrath, P. 1984. *Hags and Heroes: A Feminist Approach to Jungian Psychotherapy with Couples.* Toronto: Inner City.

———. 1993. *You're Not What I Expected: Learning to Love the Opposite Sex.* New York: Morrow.

***Polly Young-Eisendrath** is a psychologist and Jungian psychoanalyst practicing in Burlington, Vermont. Clinical Associate Professor of Psychiatry at the University of Vermont Medical College, she has published eight books, many chapters and articles, and lectures widely on topics of resilience, women's development, couple relationship, and the interface of contemporary psychoanalysis and spirituality. Her most recent book,* The Gifts of Suffering, *1996, is published by Addison-Wesley and her next two books,* The Cambridge Companion to Jung *(edited with Terence Dawson, Cambridge University Press) and* Gender and Desire *(Texas A & M University Press) will appear in the spring of 1997.*

The Pattern of Envy and Sibling Rivalry in Myth and Religion

Murray Stein, Ph.D.

Conceptualizing Envy

In a searching and vividly written work entitled *Mal Occhio*, Lawrence DiStasi recalls the tactics used by his Italian grandparents to guard against the influence of the "evil eye." He notes especially their avoidance of boasting to strangers about their children, for fear of stimulating envy. Children were so highly prized that they became the chief targets for envy attacks. Should a child become suddenly and unaccountably ill, the workings of *mal occhio* were instantly suspected, and a counter-sorcerer would be enlisted to speak some healing incantations to overcome the sickening effects of the evil eye's attack.

DiStasi does not comment on how envy attacks were avoided within the family among siblings. Some of the nastiest envy attacks take place within the supposedly cozy sanctuaries of immediate and extended family networks. For it is not only the stranger whom one envies, but the brother, the sister, and the cousin. Envy is the root of the most malignant and chronic forms of sibling rivalry.

When considering the psychology of envy, it is important to note that as in DiStasi's account, where children were the most frequent targets of envy within his culture, it is the object or quality of highest worth that draws the evil eye of envy to itself. A child will draw the attention of an evil eye in a particular setting, for example, because children symbolize the highest value there: They are the "treasure hard to attain." With this realization we can understand that envy is fundamentally based on a person's frustrated desire for direct access to the fountainhead of value, which in Jungian psychology is known as the Self.

It may seem puzzling at first to conceive of envy as being driven by the ego's deprivation of and longing for the Self, since both ego and Self are lodged in the same person and make up a single psychological unit. Yet it does seem to be the case that this is what envy most essentially is. The English word "envy," which is a derivative of the Latin *invidere*, means at root "to look into" something with intense hostility. The eye becomes hostile in this fashion when it rests upon an object that enjoys the grace of self-hood, if that same blessing is not felt inwardly as one's own inheritance too.

The envious person casts a hostile glance in the direction of a favored one and feels, at the same time, that an impossible distance lies between here and that circle of privilege and fortune. What the envious eye sees is a "selfobject" (to use Kohut's term) that cannot be brought close or enjoyed in relationship, but rather one that unrelentingly deprives oneself of grace and worth simply by virtue of its continuing existence. The graced person appears to be withholding this treasure and to want to hoard all the glory. The inner void that is hewn out and maintained by envy, which Fordham calls a "no-breast" state (199), is the breeding ground for the hatred and destructiveness so central to envy's energy. It is the ego's alienation from a Self perceived externally in projected form that creates the profound despair and deadly malevolence found in classic examples of envy's ravages, such as in Shakespeare's Iago. Envy is the alarm signal of a deep rupture in the ego-Self axis.

Envy's corrosiveness "denudes"' (Bion's phrase, 47) the inner world by destroying the site of an inwardly felt self-center. Self-energies and selfobjects, which constitute a wellspring of self-esteem and resilience when they are internally available to a person, are, in the condition of envy, perceived as being located outside of oneself, withdrawn and withholding. Thus envy is fueled by an over-investment of value in others and by a concomitant under-investment in oneself. In this state a person becomes emptied of value and resource, and the ego's total charge of energy comes to be concentrated and aggressively dispatched through *mal occhio*, the evil eye.

The Literature on Envy

In researching for this essay I embarrassed myself by falling personally into considerable envy of those who have written previously on this subject. At times this nearly paralyzed me, generating the very states articulated in the literature: emptiness, inadequacy, and excitement in the presence of the envied object. Gradually this reaction became transformed, fortunately, and I can now feel admiration and gratitude for the painstaking and insightful work done by those who have previously ventured into this rich but tortured emotional territory before me.

After its remarkable introduction by Freud in his frequent discussions of penis envy, the thread of envy in the psychoanalytic literature was picked up by Melanie Klein, who shifted the focus of envy from the penis to the breast. But beyond merely changing the focus of envy, Klein argued that primary envy is innate in humans, and she linked it to *thanatos*, the death instinct. Both females and males are born with a specific amount of primary envy, based on the strength of the death instinct in them. How the impulses of the death instinct are handled and deployed is the story of later development, but at the point of birth each of us inherits, like original sin, the capacity and the proclivity to fall into envy.

This even-handed approach with regard to gender continues in Klein's account of infancy. Since both little males and little females are nursed by a female mother, who blesses or denies them with her breast, the breast becomes the first and remains the primary object around which the emotions of love and hate swirl.

Klein's account of how envy operates in infancy and later in life is seminal to later writings by Freudians and some Jungians as well, whether these authors agree with, reject, or ignore her premise of a death instinct. In her paper "Envy and Gratitude," which has become a classic in the field, Klein makes an analytical distinction between envy and jealousy. This distinction is important to keep in mind when thinking about sibling rivalry, because sibling rivalry long outlives childhood and parents, and often has nothing to do with winning or losing the love of a third person. Envy has its proper location, according to Klein's analysis, in a two-person relationship—primordially within the mother-infant dyad, whereas jealousy is a phenomenon of three-person triangles, classically constellated within the Oedipal relationship. Envy is therefore "pre-Oedipal" and based on the feeling that the other person (originally the mother) has something good to give (a breast) but is withholding it for her own enjoyment. Her withholding of the good object is what generates envy and then also hatred of the mother. When mother is seen as reserving her goodness for herself, this perception generates the wish to harm and spoil the mother's withheld breast.

Jealousy, on the other hand, erupts when it is discovered that someone else (the father or a sibling) is enjoying the desired object instead of oneself. Jealousy drives a person to destroy the rival, so that one can have the loved object for oneself but not to destroy the object itself. In some instances of sibling rivalry it is clearly jealousy that motivates the conflict. In the most virulent forms, however, the issue has little to do with satisfying oneself by gaining the ownership of someone or something, but rather revolves around the wish to harm or destroy the envied other as an end in itself. The existence of a fought-over object—a family business, for example—only forms the excuse to face off against the envied sibling. The real wish is to destroy the envied person.

Greed, the third Fury in this shadow trinity analyzed by Klein, is closely linked to envy: it is the urgent desire to have more than one can possibly use and enjoy, to have it all (to devour the whole breast), to control and possess it completely. Both envy and greed aim for the destruction of the desired object: envy by spoiling the goodness of the loved object with one's own badness through projecting the bad parts of the self into the other (projective identification); greed by introjecting all of the other into oneself.

In Klein's view, the mother's breast is the original love object around which all of these dark emotions swirl. The breast is the source of life and therefore also symbolizes creativity itself. Klein believes that the ultimate issue encountered wherever envy appears is creativity. Having access to creativity and to the wellspring of creative energy is what envy is finally all about. From the beginning, the infant's own potential creativity is projected onto the mother's breast, creativity which the ego will need for its own growth and future integrity. Because the first vision of creativity is thus located outside of oneself, one feels dependent upon it for growth and life itself. Thus the nascent ego is alienated at the very outset from its own source of psychic creativity and growth. This must eventually be recovered by the individual psyche through re-introjection, for as Klein conceives of development, "the mother's breast forms the core of the ego and vitally contributes to its growth and integration" (215). Ego development is made up, then, of these two movements: projection of the Self into the other, followed by introjection of it back into the ego.

In her discussion of the centrality of the breast for creativity, integrity, and ego development, Klein is clearly referring to the same entity that Jung called the Self, the principal organizing archetype of the psyche, even if their descriptions and conceptualizations are very different. While Klein's discussion is object oriented, Jung's is intrapsychic. For Jung, the Kleinian breast would be taken as a symbol of the Self, a mandala with a clearly defined center. An object or image becomes a symbol when it mediates energy between the ego and an archetype, and the breast is such an object/image. The archetype that the breast mediates is the Self, which, according to Jung's later work, constitutes the core of the ego and promotes its growth and integration throughout life. The Jungian critique of Klein is that she locates the inside outside: the reason the breast has such centrality and power is that it carries a projection of the Self.

It is the absent Self, therefore, that is fundamentally at issue in the projective and introjective fantasies of the envious and greedy. Jung could easily join Klein in saying that the issue of envy is the location of creativity, but they would disagree on where psychic creativity originates and is sourced.

In a Jungian theory of envy, we would think of envy as a psychic symptom rather than as an expression of primary destructiveness, death wish, or evil. The arousal of envy is a signal of something being wrong, but it grows out of an otherwise benign hunger for full selfhood. Once constellated, however, envy can become chronic, and it can then ally itself with the shadow side of the self. At that point envy has the capacity to channel the energy of individuation (the drive toward wholeness) into destructiveness. This is the tragedy of envy. It is the story of Iago destroying Othello not to gain Desdemona for himself or to take Othello's place in the kingdom, but as an end in itself.

The insight that creativity is the fundamental issue in the problem of envy, while admitted by Klein, is not developed to any great extent in her work, due perhaps to her linking envy with *thanatos*. The Jungian authors who follow her, on the other hand, tend to take this other path. The connection between envy and creativity was picked up and elaborated by the London Jungian, Michael Rosenthall. Rosenthall held that the envied object is not the breast, but rather is "a primitive image of a phallic nature. It is an object capable of excitement, orgasm, hatred, and omnipotence. It is bisexual. This image is primarily derived from the archetype of the mother" (73). In Rosenthall's view, envy has the corrosive effect of blocking the constellation of the contrasexual opposite (the anima/animus) and thereby prevents the full experience of love. With Rosenthall, the imagery has shifted from breast back to phallus, but both are symbolic of creativity. Both are rooted ultimately in the Great Mother archetype. Both are symbols of the Self. For the chronically envious person, creativity remains in and with the Great Mother, and so the development of the individual is arrested. This person has not or cannot extract him or herself from the unconscious enough to develop individuality and separateness. Envy, according to Rosenthall, is symptomatic of an arrest in psychological development, and it functions to maintain that state of psychic stagnation by blocking the constellation of the anima or animus. It is precisely the latter that is needed to lead the individual out of bondage by constellating love.

In connection with Rosenthall's observation about the object of envy, one recalls Jung's famous childhood dream of the underground phallus, which Aniela Jaffé interpreted as the earliest symbolic representation of Jung's creativity. In Jung's case, the numinous phallus did not remain locked in the realm of the Great Mother, but became available to his conscious personality and accounted for the awesome potency (and anima availability) of his mature life. Had it not been so, he could have turned into an Iago, a genius of envy due to thwarted creativity and blocked contact with the Self.

Mary Williams, another London Jungian, followed Rosenthall's ideas in an important paper on "primary envy," and developed a list of traits that characterize chronically envious patients. Chief among these are severe borderline features, the inability to accept analytic interpretations from the analytic "mother" (a rejection based on envy), and a strong tendency to attempt to reverse the relationship with the analyst so that analyst becomes the patient and vice versa. Williams focuses on the transference features of the envious person, noting the disturbance in relationship capacities. The chronically, constitutionally envious person cannot relate to another in an appropriate object-related way.

Following on these fundamental contributions, Judith Hubback related envy to Jung's shadow concept. Her work cleanly detaches envy from *thanatos* and extends the discussion to unconscious envy, highlighting the importance for analysis, in uncovering transference and countertransference dynamics, of making envy conscious. Both Hubback and Schwartz-Salant point out the crucial need to uncover the envy component in the shadow in order for further development and experience of the Self to take place. According to these two authors—and also to the Ulanovs in their extensive and impressive study of envy in *Cinderella and her Sisters*—the road to the Self paradoxically passes through the narrow gateway of unconscious envy, and unless this difficult passage is opened the ego may not be able to come into genuine inner contact with the Self. These authors would seem to support the Kleinian notion that all of us have some amount of envy and are perhaps born with it.

Envy may not be the most royal of roads to the Self, but it does seem to offer some possibility for arriving there nevertheless. The implication is that to live creatively one must become aware of the Iago personality within, otherwise the envy that is lodged in the unconscious will block the flow of energy. This line of thought provides a point of reference for problems such as "writer's block"; they may be due to the effects of unconscious envy.

The Pattern of Envy and Sibling Rivalry in Myth and Religion

The eruption of envy in sibling rivalry occurs when a sibling gains privileged access to the Self (usually via a parent's special love and attention) and becomes so identified with it—as the favorite child, the golden boy, the chosen one—in the mind of the rival that jealousy and the usual amount of normal sibling rivalry turn into envy. The heir to the Self (whether imaged as breast or phallus) can become its owner in such a way, or to such an extent, that its blessings and nourishment and enjoyment can be withheld from others. When the threesome of jealousy collapses into the twosome of envy, we come upon sibling rivalry in its most destructive form.

A myth that lies at the core of our cultural and religious heritage depicts and clarifies the pattern I am discussing. The classic rendition of this story is found in John Milton's epic poem, *Paradise Lost*. In Milton's classic re-imagination of the Genesis story, God the Father had a son who was his radiant companion, Lucifer, a leader of the hosts of heaven. But this son was ambitious, and sought unseemly power and self-aggrandizement. Eventually, Lucifer led a rebellion against the Father and was crushed by superior force. This son fell from grace. The Father had a second son, Christ. This son was obedient and willing to do exactly what his father commanded. He made himself into a servant and offered himself as a perfect sacrifice to his Father's will.

Through perfect obedience, the second son received the full blessing of the Father and became enthroned at the Father's right hand. In fact, he and the Father became one, and what this Son commands to be blessed is blessed, and where the Son withholds his blessing the Father's is also withheld.

These two brothers, Christ and Lucifer, are now eternal enemies. The elder brother's feelings toward the younger turned to envy as he saw him become fully identified with the Father and the Father with him. This deepened his destructiveness to the point of absolute evil: Lucifer became Satan and Anti-Christ. The Father supports and maintains their split-apart condition. The elder brother goes about seeking those whom he may devour; he is agonized by greed and can never be filled. He can only destroy; he cannot create.

In this myth, there is no resolution of the problem of the envious sibling, Satan. He who once was Lucifer, the light-bringer, became the Antichrist and is essentially defined by hostility and negativity. Lucifer is a representation of the Western ego's shadow. This is the image that native peoples describe when they observe the look upon the face of the rapacious, driven European.

When Milton, a Puritan Protestant and Cromwellian anti-Monarchist, retold this myth in *Paradise Lost*, however, he conjured an image of Satan that shows great vitality and even considerable emotional appeal. One does not shudder in his presence as one would in the presence of absolute evil. In fact, William Blake later commented that Milton was secretly on the side of Satan. This preference certainly reflected Blake's own psychology and his personal hatred toward the favored religious establishment in England. Both of these poets, it might be argued, felt a need to redeem thc Luciferean shadow from its identification with absolute evil.

Jung, too, in many ways took up the part of the elder son, arguing for example that the task of modern man is to integrate, consciously, the shadow of Christianity and its lofty ideals. It is clear from Jung's writings that he was trying to bridge the split between good and evil, between the ego ideal and the ego-as-real, in himself and in his patients as well as in culture at large. This would require facing up to the problem of envy in the personal and collective shadows.

Jung discusses the problem of the Father and his two hostile sons in his essay, "A Psychological Approach to the Dogma of the Trinity." There, he places this myth into the perspective of a developmental process. First, there is the stage of only the Father, which is characterized by pleromatic oneness. This is the idyll of infancy, a state of primordial oneness and unity in the mother's womb and then at her breast. As this state of unconscious wholeness breaks up and begins to differentiate, the ego emerges and the second stage begins. As the initial stage of wholeness and unity with the world (*participation mystique*) becomes disturbed and the stage of duality sets in, the ego begins to make distinctions. The distinction between mother's breast and infant occurs to consciousness—the "I" and the "not-I"— and then comes the distinction between the mother as a whole, who is in charge of the breast, and the infant. In this stage, too, the discrimination is made between good and bad (as parts of the mother initially, perhaps; her "good breast" and "bad breast," in Klein's terms), and soon follows the distinction between good and bad parts of the Self. This begins the formation of shadow images.

This second stage is inevitable, as consciousness will develop and the discrimination of elements in the world and of disparate parts of the Self must take place. But this also inaugurates tension and conflict between the opposing parts. Now there is a good child and a bad child, a good mother and a bad one. These parts conflict with one another in the child's mind. In later development, this is the conflict that rages between the persona-ego personality on the one hand and the shadow personality on the other. At the level of religious ideation and imagery, this stage of development underlies the Christ-Antichrist conflict.

Normal development of consciousness leads inevitably to the stage of duality, because in order to function adaptively human consciousness must be able to make distinctions. But this does not necessarily lead to the kind of permanent alienation that we see in the Biblical myth, which breeds chronic enmity between the two parts, the brothers, and chronic envy in the less favored one. An alternative outcome can be seen in the Greek myth of the birth of Hermes, as recounted in the Homeric Hymn to Hermes, for example, where there is sibling rivalry between the upstart Hermes and his elder brother Apollo, but where the brothers work out a relationship under the instruction of Father Zeus, and this results in an exchange of gifts and in friendship between them. Envy becomes the issue only when the rival is perceived as totally controlling and permanently preventing access to the source of creativity and value, when one is permanently "chosen" and the other is permanently disowned.

In the third phase of development as outlined by Jung (the

trinitarian stage), the duality of the second stage is transcended and harmony is restored. (This is imaged in the myth of Hermes and Apollo: they experience gratitude and they share gifts.) Now ego-consciousness is consolidated and integrity is achieved. The hostile parts are brought back together and integrated.

Here the problem with our collective Judeo-Christian mythology becomes evident. Unlike the Greek myth of Hermes and Apollo, who achieve reconciliation and brotherhood, the Biblical myth retains the image of the "bad son" (Lucifer-turned-Satan), who is never brought back and included in the heavenly realm, alongside the image of the "good son" (Christ), who sits at the right hand of the Father. According to Jung, the Holy Trinity of Christian doctrine represents only the first stage of a possible solution to the problem of duality (and envy) and can therefore be considered only a partial representation of the integrated self. It remains ideal and spiritual but lacks shadow integration.

Since the good-bad split remains so incorrigibly entrenched in our mythology, a similar structure in our personal psychology is strongly encouraged. The shadowy, envious Luciferean shadow of the Western ego, which has been constellated in our cultural history and is revealed in this myth, has yet to overcome its estrangement and be included in the self.

With this myth of an eternal split between good son and bad son and with the identification of the good son with the father/self as our common psychological background, it is not hard to understand why it is such a struggle for many of us to feel good enough without being perfect. In Christendom, the bond to the Self passes through the image of Christ, beside whom our egos look much more Luciferean than otherwise. The very perfection of Christ's goodness casts a dark shadow on ourselves by contrast. Since Christ occupies the privileged position of the Self-image and controls access to the Self—the heavenly food, the water of life, the divine nourishment for our daily lives—we are necessarily drawn to him for our creativity, hope, and self-maintenance, but then we are equally estranged from ourselves because of our imperfection. The psychological problem is that only part of our ego can identify with Christ, and the other part—the Luciferean shadow side—remains excluded and unredeemable. In this position it inevitably becomes projected outward upon others, typically upon those who threaten our access to creativity and value. Shadow carriers are simultaneously the generators of envy reactions, and envy breeds absolute hatred and contempt. For this reason we find it so easy to destroy our enemies with a good conscience: they are evil. But our envy, as Judith Hubback points out, is in the shadow and therefore is unconscious.

The Bible, in which this myth is housed, repeats with great frequency the theme of two brothers who become locked in bitter rivalry and enmity. As we know from analytic experience, recurrent themes are critically important. Something wants to become conscious and has not been able to do so. This is the envy dynamic that is constellated by the pivotal act of God when he chooses a favorite and makes a covenant that excludes the rest.

At one level of reading, the Bible is a family saga (like Thomas Mann's *Buddenbrooks*, for example) extending over many generations. Cain and Abel set the stage. The offerings of the younger brother, a shepherd, are preferred over the offerings of his elder brother, a farmer (Genesis 4:3–5). Cain endures this humiliation until sibling rivalry turns into envy and rage overcomes him. He kills his brother. Later, the family sage, Joseph—again a younger brother—is singled out by his father for special favors. Joseph flaunts his specialness and stimulates envy in his brothers, who want to kill him but at the last minute sell him into slavery instead. Once again sibling rivalry congeals into envy and leads to murderous rage. Then David, the youngest of twelve children, is singled out to be king of Israel, being elevated not only above his brothers but also over King Saul, who flies into envy-induced rages and attempts repeatedly to kill David.

Finally, there is the instance of Jesus as the "chosen," replacing Israel in this position of privilege and entitlement. In the wider context of Western history, Israel itself now becomes the displaced elder brother. As the risen Christ, Jesus offers entry by adoption into the Father's family, and those who enter by this means occupy the same position of privilege that Christ enjoys. This leaves Israel in the position of making rival claims to this place of honor as the "chosen," and so Judaism and Christianity fall into a sort of collective sibling rivalry. Each brother claims priority of relation to the Father/self. In certain instances this rivalry has transmuted into envy and led to the wish to destroy the other.

At the heart of this family story is the image of a Father who first created all earthly peoples and then chose favorites from among his many children. The presence of this willful Parent haunts the entire family chronicle.

Chosenness is perhaps the Bible's most crucial theme. God makes a covenant with his chosen ones. Everything else hinges on this fateful decision. When the Father chooses a favorite for some irrational, inexplicable reason, he sets in motion a dynamic that in turn generates jealousy, sibling rivalry, and ultimately envy and murderous attacks both upon the chosen and the unchosen. The duality that is created by this act of discrimination becomes fixed and generates in turn a severe splitting process within history. The "chosen" form a target for envy attacks because they hold a privileged position in relation to the source of creation and sustenance; the unchosen are attacked because they carry the shadow of the chosen and are seen as evil and worthless.

Sibling rivalry and envy are embedded in the fiber of our cultural and religious traditions.

Envy and Sibling Rivalry in Practice

Among those who seek psychotherapy, there is a significant group of persons who suffer from chronic envy. Often this is more unconscious than conscious at first, in the shadow rather than openly acknowledged and consciously suffered. These people are subtly identified as rejected children, as the "bad" sons or daughters. Often these are older children who were displaced in the affections of parents by younger, perhaps more talented or presentable, siblings, the "chosen" or special ones. What may have begun as sibling rivalry of the jealous variety has hardened into sibling hatred of the envy type. These people live with envy as a daily psychic reality, and consequently they have great difficulty in forming and maintaining relationships.

Sometimes the severity of their disturbance places them in the diagnostic category of borderline personality disorder, as Mary Williams already implied. Sometimes, though, the chronic envy is so well disguised and so deftly managed by ego defences that the person does not show the typical traits of the borderline personality. This person may be well adapted, with strong and capable ego functioning, yet be continually vulnerable to subtly debilitating attacks of envy. These undermine self-confidence and self-worth and create a chronic state of tension and anxiety. This person may not explode with rage, as is so typical of borderline personalities, but rather contain and compensate for the anger and hatred by overeating, heavy drinking, smoking, or overworking. In work, there is little enjoyment of success, however, because the result is always seen as second best. As one patient put it to me many times, "I am often almost it, but never quite *the one*."

When these persons are faced with their seemingly more successful counterparts, they suffer intensely. The envied ones are those in whom everyone delights, who enjoy success and a place of privilege, those upon whom the sunshine of honor and attention beams unceasingly. The envious subject is then required to contain powerful charges of hatred and destructive impulse, and these are generally channeled into some form of self-destructive behavior.

It must be stated, too, that everyone experiences occasions of envy. Envy is a universally human emotional reaction. Patients may well feel envy toward their analysts from time to time, and analysts will also feel envy towards certain patients on occasion (cf. Hubback 1988, 111). The people I am specifically referring to here, however, are chronically envious. They live in a psychic world of continuous vulnerability to envy reactions, and it becomes their central psychological task in analysis to resolve this. The project of making chronic envy conscious is the necessary precursor to working through whatever may be its causes.

Analytic observation of the chronically envious reveals a characteristic disturbance in the relation between ego and Self. It is as though the myth cited above plays itself out in their inner world. The ego has its position and its role, but it is a Luciferean one, alienated from the Self. For this ego, even if intact, there is no comfortable inner center. In going inward, this person typically enters a void or a world of tormenting self-accusations. These persons cannot effectively soothe themselves, they cannot find comfort in meditation or active imagination, and mostly they experience anxiety, low self-esteem, emptiness, and critical inner voices. If another type of figure does appear in this person's active imagination or fantasy, it becomes the object of envy; it is the preferred one, the favored, the chosen, and the ego is thrown back into feelings of rejection and worthlessness. Fantasy in this respect follows the pattern of life experience, whose origins lie in early childhood experiences of sibling rivalry. This person lives with a constant feeling of being abused and shamed. At its extreme in the borderline personality, this is a soul in hell, consigned to everlasting torment by an indifferent or hostile parent/God.

Soothing analytic words can exacerbate the pain for this type of patient, and this creates a problem for the therapist who is trained to empathize. The patient "knows" that the analyst prefers the other patients, and certainly when the analyst's world of family and friends are taken into account the patient comes in at the end of a long line of preferred others. The transference is heavily loaded with expectations of rejection and humiliation. The analyst can of course become the object of envy as well as the rejecting parent. Always the self-bearer prefers another figure, and always the ego is second (at best) or scorned and humiliated.

Here we have the psychology of someone whose shadow may well be ideal rather than repulsive in quality. The shadow consists of the repudiated parts (traits, qualities, impulses, desires) of oneself towards which one feels aversion. In these cases of chronically envious persons, paradoxically, the aversion is felt toward the qualities (and the persons who embody them) that are usually valued by society and even as well by the envious person (though secretly). The psychological function of idealization, which is usually found to be either a defence against intimacy or a lure forward to greater integration of the Self, is here turned instead into the occasion for an excruciating envy reaction. What is projected and idealized as a valuable quality is an aspect of oneself, but because of the internal structuring of the relation between ego and Self in these persons, this turns into the meaning that someone else has more of the Self, or is better—and is therefore to be envied and hated, instead of feeling that such a privileged relationship is something to which one may aspire. The projection of these idealized features of the Self onto others drives the ego away, alienates it even further, and creates the painful repetition of humiliation and isolation. The selfobject is a shadow figure to be avoided or destroyed. For this reason, these persons form relationships with idealized analysts and others that are deeply conflicted: on the one hand there is admiration, on the other hatred and a wish to destroy.

It is tragic when these persons end up feeling evil. They become identified with the outcast child who has been condemned and driven into isolation. In their isolation, they feel worthless. Then, filled with envy toward the favored ones and consequently charged up with hatred and the desire to destroy them, they come to feel that they themselves embody evil. So complete can this distortion become that it is actually a gesture of goodness and generosity on their part when they offer to commit suicide: they would be diminishing the presence of evil on earth by at least that much!

It is this person's difficult psychological task to allow the envy-driven rage and destructiveness to fully enter into consciousness and to transform its energy into the quest and the demand for self-affirmation. In making this much envy conscious, there is at the one extreme the danger of suicide or homicide; at the other, there is the possibility of redeeming the Luciferean envy-ego and forging a home for it within the order of the chosen and the acceptable. There is also the demand and the opportunity for healing the relationships with significant others that were conflicted and broken by envy attacks.

In taking this kind of person into analysis, the analyst faces the unenviable challenge of enduring the inevitable envy attacks as transference takes hold. Understandably, the analyst comes to be seen as a person who has access to an abundant supply of good things, such as nurture, love, warmth, and admiration. The analyst also has the power to give or to withhold such things from patients. Typically in these cases, the analysand will complain of feeling deprived by the analyst, who could give so much more if only he or her were more open, more willing, more "there," more generous. The silent, receptive, empathic analyst will be seen as slyly holding back and enjoying his or her own rich feelings and thoughts, unwilling to share this wealth of psychic gold with the starving patient. Furthermore, the analyst could share her or his body, but withholds that, too. Soothing interpretative words of empathy spoken from this position can irritate and further humiliate the patient. Attempts at self-disclosure, to show that the analyst too is human and suffers similar blows and pains of living, will paradoxically stimulate envy even further: the analyst is someone who can surmount such problems and is not dragged into the mire by them. Counseling admonitions or words of consolation are taken as insults, as subtle attacks that make invidious comparisons between patient and analyst. The helplessness and diminished self-confidence felt by the analyst in response to sessions with such patients serve exquisitely well the destructive purpose of the envious analysand.

The challenge for the analyst is to survive these attacks and to contain all this hostility while waiting for the Self to show its hand from another direction. The analytic relationship can become an inky alchemical bath that may remain in the *nigredo* phase for a seemingly endless period of time. Analysis is the container for this corrosive affect, and its strength will be powerfully tested by the potent discharges of envy as the inner life of pain, bitterness, and humiliation fills the sessions. But, as the alchemists said, one is to rejoice when the *nigredo* state is achieved: this is when the chronic unconscious envy can come fully into the open and be experienced consciously and directly. Only now can it become subject to possible transformation.

What needs to be transformed is the patient's hostile attitude toward his or her own hungry Luciferean ego, so that the ego-Self axis can be repaired. Greed can then be returned to its normal proportion of hunger for good things and for the Self, and envy can be reduced to a dynamic search for the Self. The "hungry, wanting, and emulating ingredient in envy" (Hubback 1988, 115) is necessary for ego growth, not only in infancy but also in later development. Thus envy takes on a prospective function by showing the way to the Self. What the envious person envies is also symbolically what he or she desires and needs for full personhood. These needs and desires are not in themselves evil; it is the despair in the hopelessness of ever obtaining them that creates hatred and destructiveness.

A woman in her early fifties, widowed, struggling with problems of being overweight and a smoker, but more deeply with lifelong issues of greed and envy that arose and were solidified in her original family and in the sibling rivalry between her and her sister, had been in analysis for several years when she dreamed that she came to my home to go to the toilet. She entered the house but came upon my teenage son in the bathroom and so was unable to use the facilities herself. The teenager then pulled a hospital curtain around himself and withdrew behind it. This dream was interpreted in light of her attempt, reflected in the previous session, to place her "bad stuff" into me and my disinclination to let her do so. She restrained herself and did not let herself go completely. She was also angry and envious of my son, who could do as he wanted in my house. Her envy attack was not fully unleashed, however, and she was able to maintain her composure and contain the affect. She commented that my distance created an atmosphere in which it was not possible to become "closer," and while this was a long-standing complaint she also recognized by now how destructive her envy could become.

In a subsequent dream she was presented with two babies by a nun. They are twins. She smiles at them, and they return the smile. She awakens happy and gratified. It was the first time she could recall that such a strong positive response had come from other dream figures. This dream, we came to realize, was an indication that a new development was underway in her ego's relation to the Self. In this dream she felt satisfied and joyful; she felt full, loved, seen, valued. In this session when she recounted this dream, she went on to tell me how much she appreciated me and our years of work together. Her eyes welled up with tears, the evidence of gratitude. She was working through her envy of me and was able to feel gratitude because she had something of her own, a smiling infant who responded to her and promised her love.

In Klein's view, the solution to envy comes about when one feels restored to the breast and can feel gratitude for being filled rather than hatred for being deprived. The experience of love becomes possible as envy diminishes. Hubback supports this clinical observation. I would only add that envy is overcome as the Self is experienced within and lived. In the dreams just mentioned, envy is being worked on. When the infants, who represent the Self, smile and give the dreamer a feeling of acceptance, the stage of duality between good and evil is transcended and a movement toward reconciliation and integration is shown to be under way.

The acid test of this reconciliation came about in the following months and years, as this courageous patient worked on healing the deeply conflicted relationships with her mother and sister. Sibling rivalry from early childhood had spoiled the relationship between the sisters, and the hardening of it into chronic envy had its motive in the mother's perceived preference for the sister. This patient was able to transform her relationship with her mother to the point where she no longer felt rejected and pushed away. It was on her initiative and repeated efforts that this healing took place. Once the mother connection was improved, she was able to take up the relationship to her envied sister. Some two or three years after she had terminated her therapy with me, while all of this was still in the early stages of process, she came in once more to tell me of the work that she had done since we stopped meeting. She reported remarkable improvement in relationships generally, but most particularly those within her immediate family. She was now in steady contact with her sister and was able to enjoy her sister's children as never before. The envy of her sister's motherhood had dissolved enough so that it no longer interfered in her relationship to her nieces and nephews.

A second example of envy resolution is indicated in the dream of a man in his forties. Envy was a life theme with him as well, and it had recently been constellated in relation to his professionally successful wife and in the transference to me. In a sense both of us were sibling rivals. He dreamed of being placed in the humiliating position of having to become the student of a much younger man. This young teacher, though less experienced than himself, enjoyed the special favor of a senior mentor. At a critical point in the dream he makes eye contact with a senior supervisor in the audience, who indicates with a nod and a smile that he recognizes the dreamer's superiority to the young teacher. An unspoken but genuine alliance is established between the senior (father) figure and the dreamer over against the younger (positive shadow) figure. This dream shows the psyche's attempt to create an alliance between the Self and the envy-prone Luciferean ego, and to shift the burden of shadow and inferiority off the ego's shoulders. Here we see an elegant statement of the self-regulation of the psyche, as it attempts to overcome envy by creating a more positive relation between ego and Self. In tandem with this, a process of establishing a strong working relationship with me in the transference was underway. The idealization of the analyst became manageable and eventually could function as a guiding thread forward to important individuation tasks: improving his professional standing by acquiring an advanced academic degree, becoming involved himself in teaching and mentoring, and increasing his earning capacity. As envy was transformed, it became the signal for individuation needs and directions.

Conclusion

The only genuine, non-defensive solution to the problem of envy is an improved ego-Self relation, in which the ego feels that it has at least equal access to the Self *vis-à-vis* other (and especially shadow, e.g., fraternal) elements. This then makes further shadow integration possible. Until this point is reached, the shadow, much too positive and idealized, cannot be approached without envy. The ego needs to feel that "I am the embodiment, the incarnation, of the Self" in this particular space-time continuum that is my body and my life. In short, we need to feel loved.

Culturally, we are heirs of a rather hostile and critical collective father complex. This may be passed on through a mother's animus or through such a father directly. But as cultural heirs of the myth of Adam and Eve, we are in the position of the disinherited and displaced, and therefore we are especially vulnerable to envy and sibling rivalry. We do not have cultural support for feeling held and contained in the generous spirit of a loving and accepting parent who adores us. Rather, we are subject to judgment and criticism, and often to the intuition that others are preferred over us. We wonder if we are among the favored, the "elect."

Many of us, too, have been raised by critical fathers, and so we raise our children with more blame than praise. It is easier and more natural for us to find fault with ourselves, with our children, with our colleagues, and with our world than to feel cause to bless and praise them and to feel gratitude. Our spirit is ridden with judgment, self-doubt and criticism, and consequently with the potential for envy toward those upon whom we project a more positive ego-Self relation.

Perhaps on the collective level the emergence of the goddess myth is an attempt to ameliorate and to rectify this problem. The goddess may be less harsh and less preferential in her treatment of siblings. Of course, there is also a danger of regression to the pre-dualistic stage here. But, for women at any rate, who find in the goddess a representation of the Self to which their egos can look for positive identity and strength, this may well be a movement toward the post-dualistic stage of development. For men, who cannot find a Self image in the goddess, this image may represent some softening of the harsh father's critique and of his preference for one over the others of his children. Ultimately, the Self image for both sexes must mirror the ego, and the ego must feel that it is embodying the Self. "I and the Father (or the Mother) are one" is a statement of the resolution that must take place in everyone. In this sense, we need all to become Christlike. Each must feel the ego to be the proper place for incarnation of the divine. All this, while not giving up the ego's independence, self-assertion, and energetic expansion into the inner and outer cosmos.

References

Bion, W. 1962. Learning from experience. In *Seven Servants*. New York: Jason Aronson, 1977.

DiStasi, L. 1981. *Mal Occhio*. Berkeley: North Point Press.

Fordham, M. 1985. *Explorations into the Self*. London: Karnac.

Hubback, J. 1988. Envy and the shadow. In *People Who Do Things to Each Other*. Wilmette: Chiron Publications.

Jaffé. A. 1972. The creative phases in Jung's life. *Spring*: 162–90.

Jung. C. G. 1942. A psychological approach to the dogma of the trinity. In *CW* 11. Princeton, N. J.: Princeton University Press, 1969.

———. 1961. *Memories, Dreams, Reflections*. New York: Vintage Books.

Klein, M. 1956. A study of envy and gratitude. In *Selected Papers of Melanie Klein*. Ed. J. Mitchell. London: Penguin Books.

Rosenthall, M. 1963. Notes on envy and the contrasexual archetype. *Journal of Analytical Psychology* 8.1.

Schwartz-Salant, N. 1982. *Narcissism and Character Transformation*. Toronto: Inner City Books.

Ulanov, A., and B. Ulanov. 1983. *Cinderella and her Sisters*. Philadelphia: Westminster Press.

Williams, M. 1974. Success and failure in analysis: primary envy and the fate of the good. In *Success and Failure in Analysis*. Ed. G. Adler. New York: Putnam's Sons, 1974.

***Murray Stein**, Ph.D. is the author of* Practicing Wholeness *and* In Midlife *and the editor of* Jungian Analysis. *He is a training analyst at the C. G. Jung Institute of Chicago.*

Coniunctio and Marriage

Ann Belford Ulanov, Ph.D, L.H.D.

We can look at marriage in terms of which archetypes it constellates and what sorts of living experiences unfold in it. We find ourselves living with and towards our partners in patterns that arrange life's problems with unmistakable emphases. We discover that certain imaginings, somewhere in the background of our lives, have had a strong hand in shaping what we do and say. The archetypes show themselves in our ordinary behavior. For example, a patriarchal and matriarchal image of married union reveals itself in the habit of each mate addressing the other in parental language, as mother or father, or worse, as Mom and Pop (Jung 1927, par. 260; Ulanov 1971, 257). Another strong archetypal image that hovers over some marriages is one of friendship, a Hansel and Gretel connection (see also Kast 1986, for further illustrations).

I want to explore very different patterns of living that may unfold in marriage, when the *coniunctio* archetype, the union of opposites, is dominant. When this archetype comes into play in the life of a couple, it carves out a space for the marriage that differs fundamentally in source and goal from a marriage undertaken for collective reasons, such as belonging to a social institution, entering a contract, providing a frame for reproduction, or dutifully conforming to convention. The space this archetype constellates differs just as much from marriages undertaken for personal reasons, such as to please our parents, to become pregnant, or to find preferment in society. In this archetypal space we do not aim to get a parent for our inner child, and yet remarkable repair may be occasioned for the child parts in us. We do not aim to get the other to change the environment for us—to raise our economic class, for example—and yet remarkable transformation occurs inside and outside us. We do not seek a guarantee of happiness ever after, yet we may live joyously together.

When the *coniunctio* archetype is active and concretely experienced by a couple, it creates a zest in the air, an excitement about being alive, real. One feels uniquely oneself, yet engaged in one of the central mysteries of life that touch the whole family, both the present day and the intergenerational one.

What is the *Coniunctio*?

The *coniunctio* archetype is associated with the image of a mating in the *vas*, the alchemical vessel, in which base elements are mixed up, added to, and worked over to transform into a stone-hard new center of being (Jung 1953, par. 218–19; von Franz, 1980, 159–60). In such a marriage, the cooking would be operating in each partner, in between them and in both together. The interpenetration, differentiation, and integration of elements in each person's psyche would be worked on, as well as the meeting and matching and mating of all these elements between them. Such a joining is intimate at a very deep level, causing radical intrapsychic changes as well as changes in the most habitual behavior. One man, for example, expressed outright astonishment to learn that a female friend changed her sleeping patterns upon marrying. He could not imagine giving up his single large bed, as she had done, to sleep with her partner in an ordinary double-bed. "But why didn't you at least get a big queen- or king sized bed!" he exclaimed. "Because I did not get married to go on as I had, but to sleep *with* this one I love," she answered.

Such a marrying is accepted by each person deep down, not as dogma, not as driven by "should" and "ought," not as imprisoning, and not maintained to satisfy functions. Rather, it is entering through a door that opens onto constantly changing patterns, so that at any time anything may happen. It is at once secure and absolutcly open for the new to come in. The archetype is by definition indeterminate, so there is no one model or stereotype of how to be married (Ulanov and Ulanov 1994, ch. 1). This is especially true when a marriage finds its dominant archetype in *coniunctio* images, for these speak of an ongoing process, joining disparate elements in many different stages and ways.

For example, the *coniunctio* image operating in a marriage helps us perceive problems and opportunities between the two people in the light of a strong question: What is the Self engineering? (Ulanov 1994). I am using the concept of the Self here to denote the whole psyche in each partner, unconscious as well as conscious, and something more as well that gives us access to a sense of absolute reality, or of God, or of what Jung calls the *unus mundus*, the whole of existence beyond us, both material and psychical. When, perhaps, we face a problem of communication, where one partner assumes the other knows what is meant without actually verbalizing it, and feels cruelly abandoned when the other fails to understand, we can see it as an issue of the necessary death (*mortificatio*) that must follow upon a lesser *coniunctio*.

The partner who expects to be understood without having to make the effort to communicate is caught in a fusion of ego and unconscious content. This is a "lesser" *coniunctio*, because the ego is contaminated with unconscious contents that need to be differentiated (Edinger 1985, 215). Nonetheless, the fused state remains a *coniunctio* because it has come about through trust. Heretofore this partner had remained mute, filled with a noxious suspicion of rejection. To assume, now, that the other follows along with one implicitly is an achievement. Some bit of ego trusts that it is held in attention by an unconscious inner matrix and by the receptive listening of the other person. A joining, a *coniunctio*, has mended some splits in each self and in the relationship. Now much gets said, even if some sentences begin in the middle of a paragraph and meaning is left tacit.

To ask what the Self is engineering at such an impasse allows each person to acknowledge gains that have been clearly made and permits growth in this argument to keep growing. When a speaker says (or shouts) "I'm mad at you! You should understand me without me explaining everything!" then both partners can stop and ask what happens when we are not understood. They can unearth the threat of the old disintegration when one feels dropped by the other. They can join in supporting the fledgling trust that has been moving between them, but also see that something more is called for. The impasse tells them how to go further: "Speak!" it says, "speak more! Get a hold of what you want to express; I want to hear it!" The outrage on both parts signals that something bigger is trying to establish itself by busting through a joining that had already taken place. That joining is now too small. It is not content to remain at a "lesser" stage.

In the vocabulary of alchemical symbolism, this joining is too impure, the elements need to be better differentiated. As with all psychic events, so with this impasse: we find its meaning by looking back to its cause and forward to its purpose. Looking backwards, a couple can see that the lesser *coniunctio*, where each trusts the other will understand and offer a warm welcome, is not invalidated by some present difficulty. The past stands. It just is not enough. A further joining is needed, no more the old one of unconscious merger or fusion of elements in each separately, but now something new, crafted out of precise choice and with passion. Each partner wants more, not less, much more clarity about what the other wants to give and to share, which means that each must become better at finding what it is on offer and in discovering ways to receive it. The person is pulled into growth. It is work, but work with a glad ending of feeling more, not less, of oneself. The other person, the hearer, the receiver, wants to develop better hearing, stronger reception, but without being manipulated into a parental role, or, out of a misguided defensiveness, violently repudiating that role as insulting. Now, the incomplete elements of the former conjunction can be allowed to perish as both persons get to work building bigger meetings, more spacious joinings, that allow for differences between the two.

This is not to say that arguments and impasses are jolly occasions. They always bring suffering. But if we feel our suffering has purpose, that like a flower bulb breaking through a sidewalk, new life and beauty and possibility are being engineered, then we can endure the suffering and have faith in its hidden meaning.

This example illustrates a major theme in the *coniunctio* archetypal image. It joins opposites in three ways : the *complexio oppositorum*, the *coincidentia oppositorum*, and the *coniunctio oppositorum* (Jung 1959, par. 355, 423; Jung 1963, par. 176, 541–2, 662). The complexity of opposites we experience when a lot of ambivalent emotions come upon us, in opposite impulses, such as to speak, to shut up, to get mad or to accept, to repudiate or to welcome, and so on. All these parts are real enough. They fall upon us and whiz between us in great turmoil. Like Cinderella, we need to sort our seeds.

The coincidence of opposites feels more familiar: the same pairs of reactions keep turning up. We have been here before in this same impasse; I wait to hear what you mean and you wait for me to guess it, to know it intuitively. The opposites still crowd in, but now we discern some order, recall how it was before, and compare it comfortably with the present siege. We have more of our own feet. This sense of recognition is immensely reassuring to arguing couples. Instead of feeling hopeless, stuck again in the same old impasse, they can see that they are engineered to arrive at this place. In fact, I might say to new couples that the first year of marriage is inevitably a time of laying out what they will be fighting about for the next decade. In any relationship worth its salt, the two will find themselves pushed to work on their most basic personality problems and the most deep issues between them, which, because they live in the world, in history, must mirror the major issues that bedevil civilization now. The work of love is to link, to connect up, to make whole, to make gracious, to make glad. Love makes space for its own flowing from surface to depths, from each to other and back again, planting the world, making it bloom, building a bridge that extends beyond the grave. Anneliese Aumüller, the late Jungian analyst, quotes from Jean Gebser: "People who believe that there is pure coincidence lose their lives to meaninglessness. Each so-called coincidence adds to the exhilarating meaningfulness and inexhaustible richness of our lives, by making it more obvious that we are participants in the whole." (Aumüller 1963, 190).

The conjunction of opposites arrives at a union of the different elements within each person, as well as a union between them that supports each in being entirely his or her own true self. In some miraculous way, enough room exists for every element within each person to be included and none to be compromised. This comes about by a mysterious alchemy: we hold our own ground, but also differentiate it from contaminating elements and find ways to relate even to them, instead of either repressing them or falling into identification with them.

In the example above, the partner who expected to be understood without fully saying what was intended was still living in what for an adult is a contaminated state, reduced to the role of child relying on its mother. The other partner might in fact have a mother complex and slip only too easily into that role, or feel indignant that any mothering is demanded. Each person, then, must differentiate ego from threatening complex—the one to be a child, the other to be mother. If they play out those roles of mother-child, either through endorsement or repudiation, they remain contaminated, in themselves and in relation to each other. Sometimes the complex of the one partner can tell when the other is slipping into the child role again. How? Because, one can say, I feel the compulsion to be motherly. To see one's complex and hold it, rather than falling into identification with it, is to decontaminate it. It is now only a part of me; it does not rule me or my relationship. This intercession of consciousness, curiously, makes space both for the complex and for transcending it (Ulanov and Ulanov 1975, ch. 11). It is part of the "me" I bring to union with the other, but I bring it now; it does not bring me. Thus, the *coniunctio* stage does not mean each partner is perfect. But now we bring ourselves to each other instead of being driven against each other by compulsive behavior. And we find we can do paradoxical things. Our ego exerts itself to the fullest to work through problems with our partner and yet we know that the ego is not going to fix things. In the spirit of the I Ching's *Wu Wei*, we know a "Doing nothing, but also a not doing nothing."(Aumüller 1963, 192).

The complexity, coincidence and conjunction of opposites occurs over and over again in a lively marriage. It is the process by which persons go on becoming their truest selves, responding to what is fished up from the unconscious in each separately, and to what gets dredged up between them. They see all of this, sort it out, work with their own and each other's projections and introjections, and learn to unfold in relation to the objects that thus come more clearly into view. Slowly, egos become purged of possessive and power motives, what Augustine called *cupiditas*, an inordinate self-seeking, an aggrandizing compulsion to get, get, get, an unchecked appetitiveness gone wild. Paradoxically, our ego becomes increasingly dis-identified but also fat and full, living a full life. Because our ego is empty, life can gush through it with all its juices.

This process of dealing with opposites over and over again in many different patterns forms a marriage very different from the one Jung described—and Bion after him—between one partner who acts as the container of the relationship and the other partner who is contained in it (Jung 1931, par. 331–4; Bion 1970, ch. 7). Winnicott sums up the problem of the patterns of container and contained when he says:

> *[N]ot all married couples feel they can be creative as well as married.* One or the other of the two finds himself or herself involved in a process which could end in one living in a world which is really created by the other. . . . The whole problem may, for instance, be hidden under a couple of decades of child-rearing and emerge as a mid-life crisis." (1970, 44)

In the *coniunctio* image of marriage, each person is both container and contained, both for themselves and for each other, now in one, now in the other, sometimes both in both. This makes for fission, not fusion; for fire, not boredom. In the *coniunctio* arrangement neither is allowed to clamp down on personal impulse for the sake of compromise with reality demands to the point where they lose access to the creative imagination in their marriage. Both seek the alive and real in themselves and in each other. This takes time, much conversation, and work. Yet it produces in each the feeling that they are contributing to the world a small example of how to be passionate and alive in a permanent relationship, imaginatively making the world. I have known such couples and their contribution is a true one. People say about being around them that it gives them hope, that it shows them an example of love in action, an incarnation of intimacy that does not cramp but expands relationship. In one case, a woman said that because of friendship with such a couple, she dared to marry again, after an unsatisfactory marriage that had ended years ago. "I saw it could be done," she said. That is the point: the *coniunctio* archetype must be *lived* and lived in the world; otherwise it is "hanging in the air." (Jung 1953, par. 559). Marriage is one way to do it.

In the *coniunctio* arrangement, the focus is on content—on the tiger, not its cage. The tiger is what goes on in each person. What is each one's life project? What news does each bring from Self country? What do they experience together pushing and pulling them toward a greater center? This is the focus of conversation, the angle from which the problems in and between them are addressed. In Jung's language, we could say that each marriage can be a means of individuation (Heisler 1970; Guggenbühl-Craig 1977).

Aggression and Repair

How then do we live in a marriage that constellates the *coniunctio* archetype? What happens? I have three examples. The first concerns what happens to aggression and the need for repair. Aggression is used in the service of love to scour away all that is not love. Each person learns to renounce fighting dirty. Both give up going after the painful spot in the other that in more tender moments had been entrusted in great confidence. Each learns to sacrifice sadistic gratification not because of "the health of the marriage requires it" or to "be mature." I have never found that such good motives meant much at a time of intense in-fighting.

The persons give up sadism, the better to get hold of its tremendous energy, to use it for purposes of pushing through to the real and the true. The grandiose motives of winning the fight or defending oneself give way to what really matters, to find the underlying issue. One partner may say, "I'm not sure I want to be in this relationship at all," and the other might hear that, hold onto the hurt, and bring its energy to explore the feeling moving round it. Such pushing takes stamina. One wants the truth, even if the truth at any given moment may be confusion and fear.

The real and the true are the best in each, and what the Self moves into place. The best self does not mean a perfect self, but one just including all the parts, negative and doubting, angry and forlorn, as well as hopeful and enthusiastic. How to see that? How to discern the right direction? How to see where one may be caught in an old complex and where one might slip loose from it? How to know when to be silent and when to persist? These questions too, take great energy, especially if we seek our answers in a rhythm of living rather than in adherence to rules. We need aggression to focus on the true worth of the other, to dig it out, to work to restore it, and to differentiate that effort from trying to impose our image on the other.

Why should we go to all this trouble, all this work of love? Simple: Because this other, both so dear to us and so maddening at times, is made in the image of God. A transcendent presence lives in him or her. We dig down to it and excavate it. As a couple we give radical support to each other, but avoid falling into the role of therapist or parent. We each support the other's inner growth to become all the person he or she is. This includes the inner child and all the wounded and undeveloped parts as we look to repair them. But that is still not the main focus or aim. The aim is to discover what the Self is engineering. Are you listening? Will you go for it, live it, do it, love it? The support must be vigorous, summoning, lavish, and aimed right at the center of the other person's existence, in the way of the other and connected to all existence. Betrayals in marriage usually issue from betrayal of this deeper center.

Each partner fights to strip the other of false living, of pretense and half-truths, of posings and mopings. Each fights for the full being of the other, which includes the full contrasexuality of the other. We assert this sexual polarity in the other and fight against the symbiosis that occurs when each unloads the opposite sexual pole onto the partner (Ulanov 1971, 259, 296–302). How then can each of us accommodate the mixture of perceiving masculine and feminine ways of doing things, perceiving the world and acting in it, of knowing about it in ourselves? By reaching to the archetypal level of anima and animus, to see how the marriage between them opens to the indeterminacy of the archetype and steers us clear of the entrapping security of the stereotype. There is no premium put on the husband's doing the so-called masculine things, or the wife's enacting all the feminine roles. Nor do we follow, with a legalistic precision, a marriage contract which allots so much of each kind of task to each partner as guarantor of equality of chores and responsibilities. Both of us must reckon with two modes of being human in ourselves, and find ways to live with a partner who is struggling to do the same. The carrying of tasks can then be decided on the basis of personal aptitude and preference. Where both hate the same task, they do the wretched thing together—for example, one couple did the laundry at ten o'clock at night. Both hated it and put it off until they could finally face it together.

Once we understand that aggression is the means through which we secure the energy of living support, we can dig into each other, salute each other, witness each other's conversation with the Self, and fight through to the truth of each other. Aggression is repaired. No longer is the goal to see who wins or loses, who struck the keenest blow, whose defenses were the best. We aim to use our aggression to explore, unearth, pursue, receive, sustain, and support the best in each other. Our aggression works to clear away impediments, tangles and snarls, interfering blows that obstruct, block, bury, and divert us from our main concern, from the sources of our loving strengths.

This does not mean we are not wounded. Of course we are. Of course we hate fighting. But we begin now, separately and together, to see that our fighting can lead somewhere. We have excavated some old hurts and healed them—together. We have finished with some vexing issues. We have opened up new channels. This brings hope and an end to our fearful despair that aggression can only be destructive. We know now that aggression can serve love as well as destroy it.

Ruthlessness and Creativity

Ruthlessness is something most of us fear as grossly self-indulgent and abusive. It feels irrational. It is too easily confused with the violence of spouse-beating. Nonetheless, ruthlessness, as I use the word here, is a fine, strong, positive part of a marriage arranged along the patterns of the coniunctio archetype. Ruthlessness, in this sense, belongs to a person with a developed ego that is not drawn into and lost in the unconscious, as would be the case with a spouse-beater, for example. It belongs to an adult who has not given away too much of primordial aggression and sexuality. Such a person retains the capacity we see in children of going right at an object, in moves backed by instinct. For instance, a child opening a present and discovering a stuffed bear hiding in the tissue paper does not refuse the gift by doubting that this really is a bear: "Really for me? No, no: I had better not take it." The child does not reason this way, but goes right at it; it picks up the bear, nuzzles its nose, fingers its fur, loves it, eats it, chews it. We think a child is being its own true healthy self when it behaves this way. We applaud it and feel glad for it. We delight to find just the right bear for the child to unfold his or her self in such lavish use.

This ruthless love of a bear is what Winnicott calls using an object instead of merely relating to it. A child is moved by its own instinct toward an object and in unfolding itself in relation to the object (1968, 233–5; 1971, 89–90; see also, Bollas 1991, 26). The child is not at this moment concerned with protecting the object from instinctual assault or with the consequences to the object or even to its own self. The child is not trying to harm or destroy the object, but rather to use it for instinctual gratification. If the consequences turn out to be dire—if, for example, a nursing mother bursts into tears when her child bites her breast and communicates that she has been destroyed by this attack—then the child may out of love for the mother withhold such impulses toward lusty eating. On the other hand, a mother might yell, "Ouch!" and remove the offending teeth momentarily, but at the same time convey recognition, and even pleasure that the child's teeth have arrived and that such excited eating can occur because she, the mother, knows how to protect her breast. A baby can then hold onto the pleasure of instinct without diverting energy to control it by repression or dissociation, because the mother knows how to survive out of herself, not because the child has spared her. This primitive display Winnicott calls love admixed with aggression (1958, 22). I call it love with teeth.

A marriage patterned after a *coniunctio* image is one where love has teeth, with profound impact for a couple's imagination and creativity. It connects with a pair's aggression given over to the service of love. For when we allow ourselves and our partners moments of ruthless interaction, we are no longer concerned to protect them from the full force of our being all of who we are, or the full force of our energy. We do not whittle ourselves down to what we think are appropriate' proportions so that we will not threaten, intimidate, overwhelm, or hurt each other. We just are ourselves, and trust the other to be the same way. As a result, there are joyous interchanges and noisy ones and some of profound stillness, where two—each of whom is really other to the other—really meet. As if we were animals, we see stepping into the forest's clearing another animal of the same stripe and fur (Ulanov, 1986). We meet our mate.

This psychic move changes our fantasy and deepens our creativity. When each of us risks being other to our partner, in such moments of ruthless expression, we take risks. On an unconscious level, we destroy our projected image of the other. We let each other fend for ourselves. We do not seek control through projected images of who we want the other to be, or fear, or need the other to be, or think the other needs us to be. We let be. And we discover or uncover or greet the one who is left after our projections have been destroyed. The other is more than we thought, still standing there after we have given up on getting our way. We greet the freshness in otherness. Still on an unconscious level, we renounce omnipotent fantasy that would style reality according to our wishes, and discover what Winnicott calls the real externality of the other, who lives from an independent subjectivity (1971, 88–90). This may happen when the other disappoints us: he or she fails to live up to our idealized image and the image is destroyed. Thereby we release ourselves and the other to find out who actually is there. If we are using our aggression to reach the best self of the other, this is all gain, no loss; it is a scouring away to reveal the real. We may have lost a fantasy but we have gained a reality with which to interact and in which to unfold our own self. The fantasy that went into trying omnipotently to control the world, is released now to perceive the world imaginatively.

We see this clearly in the sexual arena. There, the more "teeth" our loving has, the more vigorous, variable, and pleasurable sexual congress will be. While engaging and attending to each other's needs, the two may also move into mixtures of the conscious and unconscious that allow each the freedom to drive toward climax. This is not neglect of the partner but joining on a level of ruthlessness that increases erotic intensity (Bollas 1991, 27). If too much of the ruthless element is split off, the couple may fall into a mere helping mode with each other, a sort of Hansel and Gretel cuddling and soothing that lacks sexual tone, or one person may simply service the other, who will then feel guilty for taking satisfaction at the expense of the partner, who in turn may be tempted into feelings of martyrdom. In extreme instances, ruthlessness may become dissociated and acted out in scenarios of perpetrator and accomplice (see Khan 1979, 22–3).

When we let ourselves go with all that we feel and meet up against the other doing the same, a sense of immediacy develops. We see the other with a startling freshness. We feel amazement before that familiar partner of so many years: Who is this? Who is this other coming toward me? This is how I understand the shift from omnipotent fantasy to creative imagination. The plans and preconceptions about who I am and who the other is and who we are together as a couple are momentarily wiped out in my amazement before the otherness of this one who stands before me. Like Heidegger's notion of being thrown into *dasein*, into being human—something that at any moment may go out of existence—all that I have known and been is destroyed, even if only unconsciously. This moment now is all there is, and all there is to live confronts me now, in this moment. Such immediacy brings a tremendous creative freshness to living. One is called into presence, to be all there, right now, for there may be nothing else. Right here and now, one seizes, receives, takes, and yields. Life becomes exciting and new. We are never sure about exactly what will happen.

This destroying in unconscious fantasy is like the cleansing in alchemical operations, where over and over again elements are submitted to fire, to water, to separation, to calcification, to washing and purifying. This renews us in the midst of the familiar, and makes us cherish the familiar instead of treating it with contempt. For passion to persist within a permanent relationship, boredom must be destroyed. It is automatically purged when in unconscious fantasy we dissolve the projections upon our relationship to discover its external reality afresh. Unburdened by stultifying knowledge, we come to each meeting with a sense of discovery. Newness, excitement, surprise come into our ordinary days. We claim both our imaginings and the actual reality of the other. To newness is added moreness.

Joy and the World

The newness and moreness bring joy, even in the midst of toil and stress. Stress and joy are simply two more opposites to get mixed, to coincide and unite. The hardships of living join the sense of fun that arises from keen interest in what the Self has been working in us. The goal is no longer linear, looking to arrive at a certain point and then to lie back forever after. The journey is circular, in alchemical terms, circumambulating around a center, so that the center glows and radiates its presence and energy into every little cranny, into each little misery and wounded place until every part of us individually and together is caught up in its energy and presence.

This sense of presence and liveliness creates an atmosphere of serious play, as with children. A marriage patterned around the *coniunctio* archetype provides a space for play with firm boundaries and enough room for real play. The two persons are really in it, not threatening divorce all the time, or collapsing the space of exploration by citing rules that require them always to stay together. That is looking to the cage, instead of to the tiger. The tiger is always circling around the crucial question: What is the Self engineering?

The engineering becomes complex, then, for each partner brings both a conscious ego part of themselves and an unconscious contrasexual part to the other. There are at least four presences to deal with now, and the four may at any time multiply into further relationships: ego to ego, animus to anima, then one person's ego to the other's anima or animus, and within each person, ego to contrasexual part. Crowds! Conversation whizzes along among these parts in every sexual meeting, in every fight, in every encounter. A couple aware of all these participants has much more elbow room in a fight and much more possibility of play in times of calm. For example, a woman can recognize that familiar screech of animus pitch in an argument, and may even take time out to put herself in better touch with this other force in herself in order to place the animus energy behind, not in front of her ego, so that she can better say what lies heavily on her heart. Or she may actively call on this animus energy to help her patiently penetrate the fog surrounding her mate, holding to her determination to reach him and not be put off by his mopings and sulks.

In sexual encounters, when the anima and animus as unconscious elements mix with the conscious tenderness of two people seeking comfort and pleasure with each other, their sexual meetings make space for impersonal sexual elements, even a touch of the ruthlessness discussed above, to ignite and be housed by a personal caring, each for the other. This imbues sexuality with freshness and opens it to a long range growing around a center that mysteriously combines spiritual and sensual elements. Familiarity with these mixtures of the conscious and unconscious, and personal and impersonal sexual energies, allows for much more play. The two come to know multiple exchanges of roles, relating ego to ego, animus to anima, ego to anima or animus, and even transferrals, person to person of egos and contrasexual parts. She may become the beast and he the beauty; she, the hero and he the trapped royalty, and just as quickly he the nurturing earth and she the lightning sky; he the disseminating energy and she the enfolding dark. The complexity of opposite parts is welcomed, their coincidence applauded, the conjunction understood always as a mysterious, powerful, joyous event.

Living a marriage in relation to the *coniunctio* archetype works remarkable changes in our experience of suffering too. The marriage becomes an entry point for all or any of the sufferings and the blessings of the world. Mutual penetration on conscious and unconscious levels reaches back into generations of a family and effects changes in its legacy of complexes. For example, the contamination of unconscious animus opinions about men—they are just "like that," meaning they are drinkers, or live unexamined lives, or are full of temper, whatever the accumulated ancestral experience has been—may come to a full stop with this daughter in her marriage because her man penetrates that set of assumptions and fills the space left in their wake with different living patterns. Or, on the other side, the anima premise that women properly belong in secondary roles may be upset and then discarded by the full ego life of a woman caught up in the excitement of her own projects, enlarged by her love of her mate. Not only are the ancient prejudices shaken up and made more fluid in the living experience of this couple, but something sharply different comes to replace the stereotypes which the inherited prejudices mirrored. The two persons feel they are building a new space, a new shared reality, where roles are more comfortably exchangeable because loving is more intense.

In terms of their own personal suffering, the two partners may be surprised to learn how closely their wounds match, forming still another *coniunctio* pattern. For example, a woman plagued with anxiety who needed more aggression to throw off some of the self-blame to see where faults might be located outside herself, discovered that under her mate's opposing tendency to cast blame upon others, and always aggressively assert his own stance, was a man as anxious as she! He dealt with anxiety with anger; she, with self-doubt. This insight cleared away a lot of the brush when they fought with each other, but it also brought them closer as fellow-sufferers who could learn something from each other about how to deal with the anxieties that afflicted them both.

In all these examples, the common thread is the building up of new spaces, and new realities. In alchemical terms, this is the lapis, the city, the mandala, the gold of everyday life. Oriented to what the Self is engineering, the two persons rescue and promote what is original in each other, develop faith in the unique presence of the other, both supporting it and unfolding their own uniqueness in relation to it. Thus is the new brought about; we do not "settle into the married years, " but instead feel our time together is too short! One woman reported she was astonished to hear her answer shot back from inside her to a man asking how long she had been married: "Not long enough!" And this was after twenty years.

The reason for this joyous excitement, I believe, is that the goal pictured in *coniunctio* symbolism is to reach an incomprehensible core and to live it, not to "know about it." A couple plays with the combinations of opposites flowing between them, with each in the presence of the gravitational pulls of the Self, to assemble being around the center it provides; and thus to build a new psychic structure which can promulgate new contents into consciousness. This *coniunctio* is what distinguishes creative work, where we discover the new with creative insight into ourselves or the world around us. Here, the world is our marriage. The play of masculine and feminine opposites between two of us makes a universe for true relationship.

It cannot be a relationship apart from the world. It must pull the world in and pull the two persons into the world. Why this is so has to do with the center that goes on being constructed. That core of freedom keeps producing new forms of itself that insist on going out to others and pulling others into it. In alchemical terms, the conjunction of opposites produces the lapis stone. Flowers spring up around it (Edinger 1985, 220). The mysterious center that the lapis symbolizes has a contagious effect. It gives life to all. It multiplies itself in others. It lends zest to the air. This is the greater *coniunctio*, that does not break down but breaks through the bounds of our ordinary perceiving in time and space to the presence of the beyond.

The cause and effect of the conjunction of opposites is love, a love in time and outside time. Behind the concreteness of the marriage of two people in the twentieth century stand the ancient symbols of the mystical marriage of a royal king and queen, of Sol and Luna, of Yahweh and Israel, of Christ and the Church. To be aware of this dimension is directly to participate in mystery: this is a *coniunctio* in everyday life. As Jung says:

> Whatever the learned interpretation may be of the sentence "God is love," the words affirm the *complexio oppositorum* of the Godhead.

In his medical experience, he says, he has never been able to explain the mystery of love:

> Being a part, man cannot grasp the whole. He is at its mercy. He may assent to it, or rebel against it; but he is always caught up by it and enclosed within it. He is dependent upon it and sustained by it. Love is his light and his darkness, whose end he cannot see. . . . If he possesses a grain of wisdom, he will lay down his arms and name the unknown by the more unknown, *ignotum per ignotius*—that is, by the name of God. (Jung 1963a, 353–4)

References

Aumüller, A. 1963. Personal stimulus of Jung. *Contact with Jung.* Ed. M. Fordham. Philadelphia: J. B. Lippincott Co.

Bion, W. R. 1970. *Attention and Interpretation.* London: Tavistock.

Bollas, C. 1991. *Forces of Destiny: Psychoanalysis and the Human Idiom.* London: Free Association Press.

Edinger, E. F. 1985. *Anatomy of the Psyche.* La Salle, Ill.: Open Court, 1985.

Guggenbühl-Craig, A. 1977. *Marriage: Dead or Alive.* Tr. Murray Stein. Zürich: Spring.

Heisler, V. 1970. Individuation through marriage. *Psychological Perspectives* 1.

Jung, C. G. 1927. Woman in Europe. In *CW* 10. New York: Pantheon, 1964.

———. 1931. Marriage as a Psychological Relationship. *CW* 17. New York: Pantheon, 1954.

———. 1953. *Psychology and Alchemy. CW* 12. New York: Pantheon.

______. 1959. Aion. *CW* 9:ii. New York: Pantheon.

______. 1963. *Mysterium Coniunctionis. CW* 14. New York: Pantheon.

______. 1963a. *Memories, Dreams, Reflections.* New York: Pantheon.

Kast, V. 1986. *The Nature of Loving.* Tr. Boris Matthews. Wilmette, Ill.: Chiron Publications.

Khan, M. Masud R. 1979. *Alienation in Perversions.* New York: International Universities Press.

Ulanov, A. B. 1971. *The Feminine in Jungian Psychology and in Christian Theology.* Evanston, Ill.: Northwestern University Press.

______. 1986. For better and for worse. *Psychoanalytic Review* 73,4.

______. 1994. Self-service. In *Cast the First Stone.* Ed. L. Ross and M. Roy. Wilmette, Ill: Chiron.

Ulanov, A. and B. Ulanov. 1975. *Religion and the Unconscious.* Louisville, Ky.: Westminster.

______. 1994. *Transforming Sexuality: The Archetypal Worlds of Anima and Animus.* Boston: Shambhala.

von Franz, M. L. 1980. Alchemy: An Introduction to the Symbolism and the Psychology.

Winnicott, D. W. 1958. Psych-analysis and the sense of guilt. *The Maturational Processes and the Facilitating Environment.* New York: International Universities Press.

______. 1968. The Use of the word "Use." *Psychoanalytic Explorations.* Ed. C. Winnicott, R. Shepherd, M. Davis. London: Karnac, 1989.

______. 1970. Living creatively. In *Home Is Where We Start From.* Ed. C. Winnicott, R. Shepherd, M. Davis. New York: Norton, 1986.

______. 1971. *Playing and Reality.* New York: Basic Books.

***Ann Belford Ulanov**, Ph.D., L.H.D. is a Jungian analyst in private practice in New York City, and the Christiane Brooks Johnson Professor of Psychiatry & Religion at Union Theological Seminary. Her most recent book is the* The Functioning Transcendent *and with her husband, Barry Ulanov,* Transforming Sexuality.

Archetypal Family Therapy

Developing a Jungian Approach to Family Therapy

Renos Papadopoulos

Introduction

The theory and practice of analytical psychology has largely been derived from and applied to the context of individual psychotherapy. Although, in recent years, there have been several developments in Jungian psychology (e.g. Papadopoulos 1992; Samuels 1985), it is curious that the central theoretical structures of the collective unconscious and of the archetypes seem to have continued to be used almost exclusively within the intrapsychic (individual) context. Yet these concepts refer essentially to organizing structures which are collectively shared. In this chapter, an attempt will be made to demonstrate how these concepts are fundamentally interactional systemic structuring principles, and how they can be applied to therapeutic work with families. It will be argued that the Jungian paradigm always had the sensitivity to address in a meaningful way both the intrapsychic and the collective realms (as well as their interrelationship) and it can, therefore, be appropriately applied to collective, transpersonal contexts, such as the family system. Other contexts might also include larger groups, communities, organizations, and institutions in the broader socio-ecology.

At the outset, one observes a paradox: there is plenty of evidence that Jung, on one hand, was aware of the status and possibilities of his theories and yet, on the other hand, he did not encourage their application to collective contexts. Indeed, these ideas are not merely latent within his writings; there is a plethora of evidence testifying to this effect.

In his autobiography, Jung (1963) mentioned several examples when in his early life he became aware of intrapsychic material being "shared" by different individuals, These were mainly in connection with his observation that his mother, like himself, also had her own No. 2 personality, i.e., the personality within herself, which was capable of comprehending one's connectedness with nature in a timeless dimension. When Jung entered psychiatry, his researches into complexes led him to at least two important discoveries in this respect: the first was when he found a striking similarity in the responses to the Word Association Experiment by pairs within the same family (1909), and the second was when he investigated how the complex of one girl "detonated . . . complexes lying dormant in her companions" leading to what could be called shared complexes (1910, par. 126).

The first example is most interesting because Jung, having made an astonishing discovery, was unable to explain it: After his associate, Dr. Emma Fürst, gave the Word Association Test to all members of twenty-four families, their responses were analyzed in the usual way and according to several criteria of cognitive structuring. The findings showed that the differences between and among the response patterns of individual members occurred in a regular and predictable fashion. Jung called this phenomenon "familial disposition." Moreover, he found that statistically, there were remarkable similarities between the patterns of responses among certain subgroupings within families. More specifically, the results showed that children's responses were more similar to their mothers' rather than their fathers' associations, and that mothers' associations were more similar to their daughters' rather than their sons' associations. The significance of these results is even greater if one appreciates that it was not the case of simple repetition of similar words by different members of the family, due to the given habits or family culture within each family. As Jung put it, "the daughter shares her mother's way of thinking, not only in her ideas but also in her form of expression" (1909, par. 1005). By discovering the "familial disposition" as well as similar patterns of logico-linguistic structuring within pairs in families, Jung, *de facto*, had discovered the intrapsychic interconnection within families as well as the various subgroupings or subsystems, thus anticipating modern family therapy. However, with the limitations of his theory at the time, Jung was unable to offer any plausible explanation for these phenomena. Instead, he struggled to fit them within the context of a psychoanalytic language and attributed them to the "determining influence" of the "emotional environment constellated during infancy" (Jung 1909, par. 1009). Jung did not pursue this research, and did not work with families again. However, one could argue that the phenomena he encountered at this stage of his life never left him; instead, they set him a task to find more appropriate ways of comprehending them. His subsequent development followed that very direction and enabled him to formulate a perspective within which the intrapsychic and collective realms interrelate meaningfully. Some examples of this perspective follow.

In the late twenties, Jung anticipated the modern preoccupation with the effects of socially prescribed roles upon the psychology of woman (1927). In the early thirties, he addressed fundamental questions concerning marriage and outlined a model suggesting that early (archetypal) determinants may play a powerful role in the choice of marital partner and in regressive marital interactions and conflicts (Jung 1931). In the aftermath of the Second World War, he extended the methodology of archetypal psychology to address social and political phenomena, and wrote a number of commentaries on the archetypal basis of the collective shadow which had seized Germany and ravaged entire communities and nations (e.g., Jung 1945; 1946a).

While Jung himself did not apply his theory explicitly to therapeutic interventions with families, it can be argued that this omission was circumstantial and did not necessarily follow from his theoretical premises. However, this attitude did not prevent him from recognizing the value of such applications. As Mindell has noted:

> Jung pointed out that it was often useful to work with the parents of a disturbed child instead of dealing with the child at all . . . . He frequently worked on children's problems by requesting growth in the surrounding adults" (1987, 13–14).

Returning to the central paradox which has been identified, it seems that a number of factors contributed to Jung's reluctance to take his theories to their logical conclusion and apply them to broader systems. While it is said that he did not personally favor working in a group context (Rychlak 1981), there were also the "political" considerations surrounding the early development of the psychoanalytic movement as well as the ideological and social climate of the early twentieth century; all these overemphasized the sanctity of the individual and rejected "collective movements" (cf. Strubel 1980). In other words, one way of grappling with this paradox is to suggest that Jung possibly neglected such direct clinical applications because he wanted to avoid giving the impression that he approved of "mass psychology" endeavors. Therefore, it seems that he threw the baby out with the bathwater: by rejecting the mass and the amorphous and destructive collective, Jung also neglected the meaningful and relating collective, i.e., the community, the communion. Another factor, of course, is that the field of family therapy has only developed and consolidated during recent decades, and Jung did not have the body of knowledge and clinical experience to support his endeavors in this direction.

Nevertheless, the essence of the Jungian theory, with its specific emphasis upon the archetypal structures that orchestrate both individual and collective psychological realities and behavior, is clearly expandable to encompass a psychodynamic theory of the family and, consequently, therapeutic application to the field of family therapy. Furthermore, others working within the Jungian paradigm have applied insights derived from archetypal psychology to various types of collective phenomena, for example, to politics (Bernstein 1992; Faber 1990; Odajnyk 1976; Samuels 1993), to social psychology (Progoff 1969), to the understanding of collective catastrophic events (Papadopoulos 1994), to therapeutic community (Stevens 1986), to the institution of marriage in western cultures (Guggenbühl-Craig 1981), to the development of a model for marital counseling (Young-Eisendrath 1984), and to interactional, group approaches (Boyd 1991; Mindell 1987; Zinkin 1994).

In tracing the origins of Archetypal Family Therapy (AFT), three interrelated, yet relatively distinct approaches appear relevant. They are outlined below in order to provide the background out of which these ideas and practices emerged. All three represent instances of extending the Jungian paradigm to apply to collective contexts and, at the same time, they constitute the broader metatheoretical framework of AFT.

Background Theoretical Considerations

Firstly, the findings of Dr. Bührmann's research: Dr. Vera Bührmann, a Jungian analyst in South Africa, investigated the therapeutic processes of indigenous African diviners and found a number of striking similarities between them and those of analytical psychology as practiced in the Western world (for example, see Bührmann 1981; 1984). Significantly, however, in Xhosa culture, these processes are conducted within the context of both the family and the community, and do not occur exclusively on an one-to-one-basis. This does not mean that the intrapsychic dimension is neglected; on the contrary, the intrapsychic is placed in the ecological context of the entire network of unconscious images operative in the community at large.

Secondly, the findings of a group of researchers at the University of Cape Town (from the mid-'70s to the mid-'80s) demonstrated the ability of Jungian principles to be extended and applied meaningfully to a variety of trans-individual contexts. For example, the Cape Town research group has applied Jungian theory to the area of marriage and the family, to the use of dreams as diagnostic indices capable of discriminating well-functioning from clinically-presenting families (Kaplan, Saayman, and Faber 1981), to an understanding of the positive role of androgyny in dual-career families (Cunningham and Saayman 1984), and to the process of divorce (Saayman, Faber, and Saayman 1988); in addition, in the field of psychotherapy, to dream analysis in a group setting (Shuttleworth-Jordan, Saayman, and Faber 1988). Central to their work was an earlier finding that the archetypal content of nocturnal dreams was positively influenced by induced waking fantasy (Faber, Saayman, and Papadopoulos 1983); this means that individual archetypal images belong to broader networks and are not exclusively individual products.

Thirdly, with regard to direct applications to family therapy, whereas the Cape Town group attempted to integrate the Jungian approach with the Problem-Centered Systems Therapy of the Family (Epstein and Bishop 1981), Papadopoulos (who by then had moved to London), felt closer to other systemic schools, especially the Milan Systemic approach (Selvini-Palazzoli et al. 1978). His work was based on his earlier theoretical investigations on the concept of the "Other" and its central position in Jung's own personal, theoretical, and clinical development (Papadopoulos 1980; 1984). Insofar as Jung's psychology of the Other forms the theoretical background to AFT, a brief examination of it is indicated.

In investigating Jung's approach to the nature of the psyche, Papadopoulos focused on the dynamics of the psyche's dissociability, and, inevitably, its dialectical interrelationship with the Other. His analysis revealed that Jung moved from an individual, intrapsychic concept of the Other to an appreciation of its broader collective meaning, extending even to its relationship with the structure of language. This represented a re-reading of the development of analytical psychology, according to which

Jung's introduction of key concepts—such as the complex, symbol and archetype, and the self in particular—were essentially understood as progressive reformulations of Jung's preoccupation with the problem of the Other. This involved the examination of issues concerning the composition of the "individual psyche" and its essential interrelationship with the "Other." In the course of Jung's own personal and theoretical development, there was a corresponding change in his definition of the "Other"; thus, Papadopoulos observed, Jung's concept of the Other changed progressively from a crude, physical, Other presence such as a stone, a fire, and a mannequin (see Jung 1963), to more sophisticated forms, such as internal aspects of psychological functioning, e.g., complexes, which then gradually encompassed more collective structures, e.g., symbols and archetypes.

Papadopoulos' analysis demonstrated that the movement in Jung's own theoretical formulation of the Other (from the first Other as the Complex "within" an individual, to the later formulations of the Other as Archetype) implied a progression in terms of increasing appreciation of a dynamic and dialectical interaction between the intrapsychic and what may be considered to be the "collective"; the collective inevitably includes the realms of mythological, linguistic, cultural, and social orders. Thus, the examination of the concept of the Other led to an appreciation of Jung's ingenious idea of interrelating the psychological world of the individual with *collective structuring principles*. This implies that a proper approach to the individuality of a person may only proceed through a deep comprehension of its interaction with the collective structures within which she or he is located. Thus, the very identity of the individual is forged in the dialectic between the various forms of trans-individual Others (e.g., other persons as well as cultural and cognitive predisposing structuring principles) in addition to the givens "within" each person.

It is important to note that Papadopoulos (1980) also examined the relationship between Jung's concept of the collective unconscious and language. This examination was done in the context of appreciating language as perhaps the ultimate Other, the collective structuring principle *par excellence*. His investigation included a discussion of the similarities between the positions of Jung and Lacan on the relationship between language and the unconscious. Both Jung, and Lacan (1968; 1977a; 1977b), give language a prominent position in their theories. More specifically, Jung's dictum that the collective unconscious is "the matrix of mythopoeic imagination" lends itself to an understanding of language, with its thematic and imagistic structures, as an inherent structuring body of typical themes, i.e., archetypal images. Lacan's dictum that "the unconscious is structured like language" should therefore not be foreign to the Jungian notion of the unconscious, especially as manifested in structured archetypal constellations. Both the Jungian and Lacanian positions on the unconscious refer to an essential structure and order, and differ therefore from the Freudian position—which tends to regard the unconscious as an amorphous mass of repressed material. In so far as Jung understood the archetypes as the source of our psychological connectedness, we may also accept that the network of archetypal images forms what could be termed the *Collective Structures of Meaning* (CSM). This meaning, of course, is not given but is immanent and potential.

Another reason why language is relevant to this subject is the place it occupies in the theory and practice of systemic family therapy, throughout its brief history. In the early days of family therapy, when there was more emphasis on communication theory (e.g., Watzslawick, Beavin, and Jackson 1967) the division between analogic and digital language was central in understanding the different messages given by family members, and how these were forming a collective structure which was underlying the individuals' own perception. Then, Shands' observation of the "tyranny of linguistic conditioning" (Shands 1971) assisted the Milan group of family therapists to develop their own explicit theory about the linearity of language, which essentially tends to impose a causalistic and deterministic perception of reality. The Milan therapists countered the tendency of linguistic determination by consciously devising non-linear (i.e., systemic or circular) therapeutic statements and interventions (Selvini-Palazzoli et al. 1980). A small detail which requires due attention (and which, however, falls outside the scope of this chapter) is the fact that Paul Watzslawick was initially trained as a Jungian analyst (he graduated from the C. G. Jung Institute in Zurich) and in the early days was invited by the Milan group of family therapists to assist them with developing their approach. To return to the theme, it seems that the role of language is crucial because it creates perhaps the most important category of the *Collective Structures of Meaning.* As Keeny characteristically wrote, "Language is an epistemological knife. It slices the world into bits and pieces, provides names, names of names, and names of names of names" (1983, 110). This should be compared with Jung's own exclamation that "it is difficult to divest conceptual language of its causalistic colouring" (1952, par. 965).

To summarize, language not only helps us appreciate the presence and texture of the collective tissue which binds individuals together but also forms a particular Collective Structure of Meaning which has a powerful influence on every single facet of our perceptions of our world, ourselves, and our very own experiences.

Metatheoretical Framework

The implementation of a Jungian approach to family therapy should not necessarily imply a mechanical transposition of the processes of individual psychotherapy to the interpersonal, systemic context of the family; while it is sensible to make use of such processes, it is important to be aware of their limitations. Moreover, it is imperative that one should endeavor to develop new insights, and processes more appropriate to working within family systems, which nevertheless should remain firmly grounded in the Jungian paradigm. For example, an archetypal approach to family therapy, similar to analytical work with individuals, elicits processes of confrontation with and integration of the shadow, e.g., images of the "trickster," the "rescuer," and so on; however, Archetypal Family Therapy focuses more on the interactive dimensions of such motifs, which have broader collective meaning. In other words, it is necessary not only to observe the archetype of the trickster as gripping one person but also to examine the impact it has on all other members of the family. Moreover, it is useful to explore with the family why, at this particular time, this particular individual incarnates the trickster; in other words, what is the function and purpose of the appearance of the trickster archetype for the whole family at this specific time. Another important consideration is the differentiation between the development of the individual in the context of (instead of in opposition to) the development of the family. For example, processes such as the "differentiation of the ego" and the "emergence of the self" refer to intrapsychic phenomena of an individual and need to be supplemented with interactional processes which, nevertheless, do not exclude the intrapsychic dimension. Therefore, one could begin to observe the differentiation of the *family ego* and of the *family self* (so to speak).

It may now be possible to begin to articulate this Jungian metatheory of family dynamics. Crucial to this would be a systematic analysis of the meaning of the archetypal hypothesis. Archetypes are not isolated entities but form interrelated structures. Clinical practice as well as theory show that archetypes are bipolar in nature and also relate to each other. For example, the positive and negative anima interrelate with the positive and negative animus within the context of close relationships. Moreover, these images also exist "outside" the individuals and thus form what could be called a systemic network. Another important aspect of the Jungian paradigm is its dialectical approach to psychotherapy (Rychlak 1984) where various archetypal principles are seen to orchestrate perceptions and behaviors between relevant others (husband/wife, mother/father, parent/child, brother/sister, and so forth) both at the intrapsychic (*subjective*) level as well as at the interpersonal (*objective*) level. The notion of archetype posits a dynamic interaction between, on one hand, collective structuring principles (*collective* patterns of behavior and their reciprocally related archetypal images) and, on the other hand, intrapsychic processes located within the individual in personal, family, group, and interpersonal, social contexts, i.e., the various dimensions of an *individual* psychosocial world.

Jung's unique contribution is his appreciation of collective structuring principles in the formation of an individual psychological world but, importantly, this is not envisaged in terms of a deterministic, causal, mechanistic, linear relationship which exists outside of an interactional, systemic context. Rather, the basic concepts are compatible with the language of modern systems theory (cf. Vetere 1987). For example, Jung compared the archetype to:

> [T]he axial system of a crystal, which, as it were, performs the crystaline [sic] structure in the mother liquid, although it has no material existence of its own . . . The representations themselves are not inherited, only the forms, and in that respect they correspond in every way to the instincts, which are also determined in form only. The existence of the instincts can no more be proved than the existence of the archetypes, so long as they do not manifest themselves concretely." (1954a, par. 155)

In essence, Jung's theory posits that the life-cycle is orchestrated by archetypal structures which manifest as potentialities at certain critical, bio-psycho-social developmental periods. The archetypal structures, although lacking inherited individual content, are actualized in and modulated by the particular circumstances of the individual's life experience in a social context which Stevens (1982) has described as "species specific." This is in accordance with the modern understanding that the human life-cycle, together with all other organic and inorganic processes, is subject to modulation by broader ecological systems. Applying these concepts to the human family system, it was noted that:

> Jung's concept of a transpersonal level of human experience suggests that dynamic unconscious processes are characterized by a commonality between individuals, and it is precisely in this sense that we understand the term "collective," in contrast to the intra-personal interpretation usually associated with the intrapsychic model. The theory of archetypal relationships, simply stated, contends that human development, seen from both phylogenetic and ontogenetic perspectives, represents a process of mutual adaptations between the sexes as well as between parents and offspring. Inherent archetypal images of the father and mother in the child, and of the child in the parents, intermingle and interfuse on an unconscious level in family interactions. The archetype is thus embedded in a nexus of mutually adapted patterns of relationship and must be understood within the context of the individual's unique socio-ecology. In the Jungian theory, therefore, intrapsychic functioning must be viewed within the framework of human social systems." (Kaplan et al. 1981, 228)

Therefore, the present approach to family therapy is informed by the theoretical understanding that dynamic, systemic and dialectical inter-relationships between the individual and the collective (the family) are mediated via archetypal images. For example, the individual is bound to experience the archetype of the father, which *necessitates* a personal experience of the father in order to develop a personalized and integrated or "individuated" form of this collective structure. Jung indeed warns of the dangers and various levels of potential pathology in those cases where this process fails to be adequately actualized. It follows, therefore, that the archetype is the impetus and potential background which must become personalized and integrated. Failure to adequately accomplish this has the result that, in the context of the family, members act in a purely collective manner, and are driven, manipulated, and coerced like puppets in an archetypal scenario to play set, predetermined, collective roles, adopting polarized, often confrontational and conflict-ridden archetypal positions such as "the bad mother," "the over-domineering father," "the eternal child," and so forth.

The archetype, therefore, as it has emerged from this discussion, is essentially a *relational*, an *interactional* concept; indeed, while Jung's predominant presentation of the archetype (and its extensive use thereafter) emphasized it as a notion almost exclusively confined to the individual, the archetype, logically and theoretically, by its very *nature*, cannot but be a relational concept. Jung, as it has been noted above, also employed the concept in the context of relating the individual to the collective. However, not only Jung himself but also the post-Jungians seem to have neglected to deal with the idea of the "collective" in its most direct, primary, and immediate form, i.e., in the individual's obvious experience of the collective, *the family*. Thus, archetypal constellations in the individual cannot be appropriately understood outside the context of the immediate network of family dynamics. For example, the archetype of the "devouring mother" presupposes that the mother has somebody to devour; moreover, the other members of the family must respond to this "devouring" in some way, either by approving or disapproving of it. In other words, this phenomenon does not happen in a vacuum but in the context of others who are directly affected and shaped by one individual's archetypal possession. Moreover, the very occurrence of this archetypal possession is not an individual event, unrelated to the other members of the family. It has a meaning, a purpose, and a function for the whole family. This means that insofar as the impact of an archetype is on the family as a unit, it is difficult to even conceptualize that thc archetypal possession is of one individual. The appropriate framework to understand such phenomena would therefore be the *network of archetypal images*; according to this, archetypal images interact with each other and with the family members as the family members incarnate them. In this way, one may say that the family, *as a unit*, manifests and works through a specific, archetypally orchestrated destiny; so much so, that Jung himself wrote that it frequently takes generations of a family to work out a certain archetypal destiny (Jung 1909).

Another theoretical implication of this formulation is that the family, as a *system*, interacts with the world in such a way that certain functions or individual roles are assigned in a non-reflective or "unconscious" manner to certain individuals. For example, when nurturing and affective family functions generally associated with the archetypal feminine principle (and, consequently prone to falling into sex-role stereotypes), are assigned to an overburdened wife in an one-sided manner, consistently and without due reflection and negotiated contractual agreement, the result is often a marital breakdown (Saayman et al. 1988). Thus, in order to maintain an overall, homeostatic family unity, an individual may be designated and destined to carry out roles which may be detrimental to him or her as an individual, but which roles have the function of compensating for other functions, trends, or archetypal dimensions in the family. This leads to an understanding that a central goal of family therapy, within a Jungian framework, is the movement away from an overall homeostatic family equation, where the balance is maintained at the cost of individual pathology and individual one-sidedness; instead, the family is facilitated to digest, in measure, the constant change of archetypal images which interact with the family. In this way, family members find, each one of them, a personal response and individualized position with regard to the particular constellation of the network of archetypal images as it is active at the time, and may avoid being players of archetypally assigned roles. This leads to a more meaningful way of interrelating, which enables reciprocal growth.

The final aspect of this framework is Jung's theory of compensation. This is a useful principle, if not taken to extreme forms, especially because it has strong systemic overtones. Jung's theory of compensation as applied to the teleological meaning of dreams (Mattoon 1978), as well as to the functions of the symptoms of neurotic and psychotic disturbances, has indeed anticipated the modern interactional understanding of the systemic function of the "presenting problem(s)." The presenting symptom often is a means to maintain a homeostatically closed family system as well as an opportunity to open the system up and change away from the symptom. Thus, Jung's understanding of the prospective (purposeful) functions of dreams and symptoms, together with the central theory of the network of archetypal images, forms a potentially comprehensive theoretical edifice, which joins a psychodynamic approach to the individual with a systems approach to family functioning. The heuristic and applied value of such an extended theory of analytical psychology, therefore, is that it may circumvent the dangers inherent in "mixing models" via an undisciplined and *ad hoc* combination of "eclectic" approaches (Epstein and Bishop 1981), since it would enable the use of one therapeutic language (metatheory) to encompass both intrapsychic and interpersonal phenomena, as well as the interface between them. This kind of metatheory may thus be capable of informing therapeutic interventions not only with individuals in an one to one analytical setting but also with individuals and other combinations of subsystems within family networks.

Key Processes

Although it is inappropriate to imply that this approach, similar to any other meaningful therapeutic intervention, can be reduced to cut-and-dried techniques and steps, nevertheless it may be useful to attempt to articulate some key processes which occur in this approach to Archetypal Family Therapy in order to strengthen the clinical dimension and facilitate better comprehension. These processes are interrelated and not exclusive of each other and do not necessarily follow the same sequential order. Finally, insofar as they represent the distillation of clinical experience of working with families, they are descriptive and should not be taken as dogmatic and prescriptive. Nevertheless, it is hoped that they could serve as useful guidelines to be used creatively.

Movement from Individual Minds to Archetypal Networks

The first process refers to the assessment of the problem(s) presented by the family. However, this assessment is not of the linear, causal type usually associated with the term "assessment." More concretely, in exploring the reasons why a family seeks assistance, the emphasis is on elucidating the contextual network of these reasons and not their static definitions. This means that the therapist is interested in the effect and impact that these "reasons" have upon the various *dramatis personae* as well as in their broader meaning, which locates that particular family within a particular archetypal *impasse.*

To begin with, families usually come to the attention of professionals as the result of a distinct problem generally perceived as located in an individual. By means of a series of successive, professional reformulations, they may be referred to a family therapist. Even at this stage, families normally continue to identify an individual as "*the cause* of the problem." At the same time, the very referring networks (with corresponding treatment implications and expectations within the framework of "the helping professions") may activate re-enactment of a number of archetypal whirlpools; this inevitably assigns designated roles to each and every member of the family as well as to the therapist(s). For example, the person who carries the symptom—the "patient" (or in family therapy terms: the index or designated person)—may be assigned the role of "bully," and the therapist that of "savior/rescuer." This sets up intrapsychic and systemic dynamics in which projections and collective expectations play a major role. It is therefore the therapist's task not only to anticipate these dynamics from the outset but also to locate him or herself within this context.

The initial therapeutic focus is therefore on developing an understanding of how the particular problems relate to the entire network of family interrelationships. This effectively means an analysis of the archetypes which orchestrate interactions and transactions in the family at intrapsychic and/or interpersonal levels. This happens when the symptom is expanded in terms of its imagistic dimensions. Language is a remarkable treasure house of images; in addition to its function as a medium of *communication* (along a linear, sign-type dimension), language *evokes*. The power to evoke is inherent in the imagistic dimension of language. As Jung put it: "Image and meaning are identical; and as the first takes shape, so the latter becomes clear" (1954b, par. 402). As perhaps the ultimate Other and one of the most important categories of the Collective Structures of Meaning, evidently, language shapes us more than we shape language. It is imperative, therefore, to connect with that Collective Structure of Meaning which had been instrumental in creating in us the very ways of perceiving what we considered as problematic. Thus, the therapist assists the family in exploring metaphorical meanings and images connected with the concrete problem and these are interrelated to connect with the network of archetypal images activated in that particular family at that time. For example, the physical act of bullying may be examined in terms of the images of forceful imposition which each one of the family members experiences in relation to external as well as internal pressures, both as a victim as well as perpetrator. In this way, it is possible to develop an additional dimension to the symptom within which all family members find themselves meaningfully interrelated among themselves as well as with the dominating images.

This development can lead to a gradual elicitation of a new way of perceiving reality, i.e., of a new and different epistemology within the family unit. This emerging epistemology would be devoid of the usual key ingredients of closed and stuck systems; the latter often include the assignment or distribution of blame, and the causalistic, linear interpretation of the source of the family difficulties, problems, and ultimately symptoms. At this stage, a gradual redefinition of the problem may already begin: instead of understanding the problem as being the sole ownership of one person, or as the consequence of the actions of one particular family member, the "problem" is appreciated as one manifestation of the overall archetypal network currently operating within the family.

More specifically, the therapist may focus on:

(a) The contextual identification of (i) the self-referring archetypes of individuals such as the persona, shadow, anima/animus, and (ii) family archetypes such as home, marital and parental relationships. The identification is achieved by means of delineating specific themes or images which appear to link characteristic patterns in the organization of the family. The exploration of these themes proceeds with reference to each individual as well as to subsystems within the family and, ultimately, to their meaning within the family as a whole.

(b) The exploration of the symptom and the identification of the corrective, teleological function latent within the presenting problems. This is a very important aspect of the process and it is directly based on Jung's appreciation of the symptom as having a corrective and thus potentially healing function. In doing this, the therapist investigates and identifies issues such as family myths, beliefs, conflicts, patterns, and roles, as manifested in characteristic interactions, repetitions, dreams, fantasies, differing versions of events, and so forth. Jung anticipated modern systemically oriented family therapists (e.g. the Milan approach) in appreciating that the "symptom" is by no means merely an obnoxious phenomenon that needs to be mechanically removed or "cured." He insisted that the therapist should examine the *meaning* of the symptom since it may suggest a solution *in potentia* and indicate a direction that, if studied appropriately, would be extremely instructive for the whole family system. This, of course, is similar also to Jung's understanding of the meaning of dreams which he viewed, not as disguised and deceptive pathological manifestations, but as useful messages from the unconscious, thus conveying the corrective intimations of some neglected and unconscious aspects of the psyche/system.

Neutrality

In working according to the above guidelines, the therapist perforce becomes neutral in her or his attitude to the family. In other words, the stance of neutrality is not an epiphenomenon; it is not an adopted attitude based on some external theoretical, ideological, or ethical system, but it is integral to a proper understanding of the dynamic networks operating in the family. For example, the therapist cannot possibly take the side of one member of the family against another or favor one "solution" rather than another, when he or she appreciates that all members of the family are parts of a collective unconscious scenario. "Neutrality," therefore, does not imply either apathy or neglect, neither "detached professional distance" nor lack of engagement with or commitment to the family. More specifically, it refers essentially to the following issues:

(i) Blame of and by individual family members.

The therapist, as far as possible, avoids taking sides within the family "blame-game," not because of an external adherence to some abstract code of ethics but because of a proper appreciation of the totality of the family network. This appreciation dictates a painstaking focus on the function and meaning of each individual attempt at blame.

(ii) Initial, one-sided "solutions" either openly suggested or implied by family members.

These may ultimately be understood as an expression of the overall existing archetypal domination. In other words, these "solutions" more often than not tend to be reactive and impulsive, and their ultimate function is to maintain the pathology of the status quo. As such, these "solutions" usually betray the very nature of the archetypal constellation which grips the family at the time. These should be distinguished from the appropriate solutions, which are a product of a genuine movement of the entire system, and a result of a genuinely new family epistemology.

(iii) Attitudes towards the symptom.

The family usually has a great investment in the removal of the symptom(s), as these alone are usually perceived as "the problem." The therapist, however, cannot afford to be unreflectingly drawn into adopting the skewed perspective which identifies one isolated aspect of the system as a symptom. Instead, she or he needs to create a climate and a different context within which the family members may risk and abandon the powerful, one-dimensional wish to remove the symptom at all cost and instead develop a curiosity to explore the meaning and function of the symptom within the totality of the family system.

Neutrality has been one of the hallmarks of the Milan Systemic Family Therapy approach (e.g., Selvini-Palazzoli et al. 1980). This approach to neutrality emphasizes the distance that the therapist needs to maintain in order to observe the system in a more methodical way. The entire practice of family therapy reflects this concern. Originally, the Milan guidelines suggested the use of two therapists in the consulting room and a team that watched the therapy session from behind an one-way mirror. The session was divided into a pre-session discussion, which included the two therapists and the team. Further, during the course of the actual therapy session, there were breaks when the observing team provided input to the therapists and, at the conclusion of the interview, there was another post-session discussion when the whole consultation was reviewed within the context of the family system plus the therapists. In this way, the Milan approach attempted to separate the system of therapists from the family system and then endeavored to observe their interaction.

It seems that all therapies have to follow the same path in the course of their development. Psychoanalysis initially attempted to keep the therapist in a sanitized position and away from the patient's world so that contamination should not occur. Thus, Freud's initial efforts were to eliminate any counter-transference (e.g., Freud 1914). It was Jung who first pointed out that counter-transference not only was not detrimental to the therapeutic process but was essential in providing the therapist with the correct information about the therapeutic dynamics (1916). Predictably, the Milan school's original position has been adjusted, and now there is due recognition of the importance of the therapist's presence; the current focus, therefore, is on the meticulous examination of how the two systems are interconnected rather than on attempting to avoid any connection between them (cf. Cronen and Pearce 1985).

Therapists, however, cannot possibly remain emotionally uninvolved, and their active immersion within the family system is essential to the dialectical therapeutic process. Archetypal Family Therapy attempts to achieve a synthesis between the neutrality outlined above and the necessary involvement of the therapist. This issue is also similar to the debate on the role of transference in individual Jungian psychotherapy (Spiegelman 1980): Are therapists "blank screens" onto which patients projects their transference, or are they actively involved in an interaction with the analysands? Jung's alchemical metaphor of therapy (1946b) renders this dilemma superfluous. Thus, rather than posing a dichotomy between the one or the other stance (Newman 1980), it is a question of finding an appropriate metaphor (e.g., the alchemical one) which permits complementary roles for both of these important processes in therapy. This issue will be re-examined further below.

Stories of Archetypal Designations

In interacting with the family, the therapist gradually encounters various stories that members of the family tell about themselves, about individual members, thus making intelligible key events in their history, the behavior of central characters, and so forth. It is important to accept these stories as stories, and not as historical accounts. There is a therapeutic skill in transforming straightforward accounts into stories. Stories move more freely in time and space and are not fixed to set conditions. Therefore, time, place, and the *dramatis personae* can be substituted. Moving in this direction, the therapist distinguishes between those features of the story which are changeable and those which are unchangeable. For example, through the family stories it may be found that in that particular family, at least one woman must always remain strong and carry the rest of the family in times of crisis; or, in another example, there will always need to be a child who will be expected to betray the family. These kinds of unchangeable features can be compared to central beams in houses which must always remain unmoved; alternations and renovations may take place as long as those central beams are kept intact. Similarly with families, some central characteristics seem to need to remain in place at all cost.

The implications of this realization, of course, is that family members are assigned designated combinations of archetypal roles, so that the family scenario ensures that the central feature(s) are retained. The stories of "central family beams" also reveal the belief systems that the family hold, which connect with the particular constellation of archetypal images operating across time. In identifying such trends, the therapist in a sense relates to what may be called *the archetypal destiny* of the family at that time.

In addition to the identification of the self-referring and family archetypal themes mentioned above, the therapist will need to appreciate his or her own position within this archetypal network and his or her own designated role in terms of the stories of "family beams." The main instrument available to the therapist in ascertaining this is his or her own countertransference. This is not an intellectual exercise based on theory. The therapist needs to almost allow her or himself to slip into a less vigilant state and then catch (so to speak) him or herself experiencing certain feelings, thoughts or reactions which should be kept in safe storage. Later, in a more self-reflective and vigilant state, the therapist examines the meaning of these responses in her or himself and connects them with the therapeutic situation. In this way, the therapist becomes aware of his or her own position within the therapeutic system.

This process is a very delicate one and the therapist needs to distinguish the overall *impact* on him or herself almost on a bodily level. This is comparable to Plaut's term "incarnation of the archetype" (1974; 1993). However, it should be clarified immediately that the use of this term is an approximation of the analytical term; in individual analytic work, an elaboration of this process requires intense, frequent sessions over a longer period of time, whereas in AFT an analogous process occurs which can be worked through within the context of less frequent therapy sessions and over a shorter period. Therefore, one should be cautious in transposing this concept to the different therapeutic context of working with families, in which there is a network of interrelationships among individuals as well as among archetypal images. Needless to say, it is not sufficient merely to identify, in a broad sense, which particular archetype the therapist is perceived to be incarnating at the time. The process is far more complicated. and one may not be able to pinpoint one specific archetype which the therapist incarnates, although it is likely that there would be an imagistic tendency pointing towards some thematic coherence. Moreover, it is essential to appreciate the implications which that particular incarnation has for the whole network of family interrelationships. In other words, the therapist observes, experiences, and articulates the reciprocal impact of this process upon both the family and the therapist.

Therapist's Dilemmas

Among the many dilemmas the therapist will face will be those in connection with accepting or rejecting the role dictated by the archetypal designation in its existing formulation. However, the alternatives are not limited to these two options. The therapist may, indeed, reverse the role. For example, if she or he is assigned the role of the "protector" by the family constellation, she or he may deem it more appropriate, on certain occasions and when necessary, to reverse the role to that of "passive observer." The differential effect which may then be created by these contrasting approaches might enable the family to appreciate, in a direct and experiential manner, the archetypal expectations that organize them as a family. Moreover, the therapist has other options. He or she may decline to enter actively into any set role, but in contrast may interact with the family from the hypothetical position of posing questions "as if" he or she were in one or other set position. The differential dialogue that will ensue upon this appreciation of the dilemma will itself lead to a different perspective within which the dilemma will no longer be experienced as necessarily intractable. In other words, the therapist's dilemma—to accept or reject the role that the "archetypal designation" dictates to him or her—will inevitably be experienced by the family as well. Thus, this dialogue will be both internal (within the therapist) as well as shared with and within the family. It may take the form of hypothetical questioning addressed to family members, such as: "If I were not to suggest ways of protecting you from your husband's anger, how would that affect your relationship with your daughter?" The important point here, accepting the hypothesis of the collective structures of meaning, is that one appreciates, in addition to the interaction at the external, interpersonal levels, that there is also another, deeper level, which derives from the impersonal and archetypal networks.

Renovations

In all renovating work there is a combination of destroying certain parts, building new ones, renovating old sections, and creating new connections and divisions among different sections of a structure. However, in all this work one cannot afford to forget the main beams! Any careless enthusiasm in rebuilding which would ignore these beams leads to disaster. One, therefore, needs always to respect the main beams; our very safety depends on them. Some of the main conflicts and ensuing tragedies in families stem from Sisyphean efforts on behalf of certain members of the family to go against these beams. Thus, the therapist's task is to find ways of creating a context where a genuine and appropriate respect of these central beams is maintained. If the therapist and/or the family adopt any other attitude towards the main beams, the results may be catastrophic. Examples of such inappropriate attitudes include fatalistic acceptance, rebellious attack, denial, a passive aggressive stance, and an inflated omnipotence towards them.

Ultimately, all therapeutic transformation needs to balance *change* with *stability*. Too much or too little of either will create unnecessary distress, which may lead to symptomatic behavior. An attitude of appropriate respect towards the power of archetypal designations facilitates the emergence of a new family epistemology, within which a respect for the stable parts of the system is supplemented with a measured need for appropriate change. Working along these lines will often lead to the emergence of new conflicts between individuals and the collective, between the family and the therapist, and between new sets of alliances. These may not necessarily be new in terms of the protagonists but may be new in terms of the content and context. On occasions like these, it would be important for the therapist to enable the family not to perceive them as a sign of deterioration of the situation; instead, they need to be understood in terms of the inevitable upheavals of renovating work.

However, as with all renovations, one needs to know the plans, and where the renovations will lead. It could be said that there are two types of therapies: on one hand, there are those which set clear therapeutic goals, e.g., the removal of certain behaviors and acquisition of new and specific ones, and, on the other hand, those therapies where the goals are less specific and are more connected with the development of new processes.

AFT, similar to the Jungian analytical work with individual clients, belongs to the second category. It could be said that the goal of both of these therapeutic approaches is the development of a new epistemology where the individual connects meaningfully with a bigger whole. Jung wrote about this process in various ways, e.g., trusting the wisdom of the unconscious, following the objective psyche, benefiting from the archetypal correction, etc. All these expressions convey a process which is identical with what occurs in AFT when individuals connect with broader systemic contexts.

Towards a "Lysis"

It is difficult to talk about a cure in modern psychotherapeutic endeavors. This does not mean that psychotherapy is not responsible for behaviors to change or that new positions—one's promising fuller growth—are not found by patients. The Greek term *lysis* seems to be an apt one to describe the complexities of therapeutic outcome. *Lysis* is the noun derived from the verb *leo* (to untie, to loosen up). Aristotle in his *Poetics* uses the noun *lysis* to refer to the end of tragedy, and in that context it means the "solution," the "resolution." However, in the same work, Aristotle contrasts it to *desis* (1965, 55b24), which means the opposite, i.e., to entangle, to tie up. Thus, *lysis* as "unraveling" appears to be a useful metaphor for therapy, where no new *dramatis personae* need to be added and no existing parts need to be chopped off. Instead, the existing materials are reshuffled in a way that the knot is disentangled and the rope is available for better use.

In unraveling a story, we free it to be reused in a different way. The story is bigger than its tragic parts, and the rope is bigger than the knot. Similarly, the individual conflicts fit in within a bigger whole, a broader archetypal scenario which does not need to be rejected because it also contains the deliverance. The new emerging epistemology of the family enables the family members to appreciate that the "system is greater than individuals" and that their own freedom or disentanglement from the system does not require its destruction. However, in a seemingly paradoxical manner, at the same time that the knot is unraveled, the system itself does change. The new family epistemology enables the family members to experience directly and experientially their interconnectedness, and thus makes the dominating power of the archetypally orchestrated impulses more manageable. Thus, each family member may increasingly be able to relate to others within the family (and outside) in a more individuated, autonomous manner, beyond the confines of the restrictive repertoire of the archetypal constellation.

This approach has parallels with Bateson's (1973) theory concerning the "power greater than self," which was illustrated by his work on alcoholism. Bateson observed that the therapeutic turn for the alcoholic occurs at the point when he "hits rock bottom" and realizes that he in fact has no control over his drinking. As long as the alcoholic believes in his ability to stop drinking, he lives with a false hope and cannot accept the fact that his drinking is bigger than him. Once he "hits rock bottom" and gives up hope, then the state of surrender which ensues allows him to develop a new epistemology within which he appreciates his relative impotence. This very realization is also his real hope for change. It is at this moment that the alcoholic may have a direct experience of the fact that his drinking is not located in himself, but that rather he is located in the broader context where his drinking is located. In other words, the system comprising the contingencies of his drinking as well as himself is bigger than his own individual "self." This realization breaks the separation between himself and "his problem" and interrelates them within a broader systemic context; this is what the new epistemology enables him to perceive, and this is likely to result in the loosening of the power of the archetypal grip.

The new family epistemology implies the "archetypal correction" of individual egos in tune with systemic contexts. In a manner reminiscent of Jungian theory, Bateson approaches the resolution of a problem via the development of a new epistemology which circumvents a causal, and one-dimensional (either intrapersonal or interpersonal) formulation. This requires the poetic appreciation that the system is more powerful than the individual, that the archetype is stronger than an individual wish, that the complex possesses us rather than our possessing the complex, and that the dream is dreaming us, rather than we dreaming the dream.

Clinical Vignette

The following short clinical vignette is intended to provide an illustration of some of the processes described above. A fuller clinical case, according to an earlier form of the AFT, is described in detail elsewhere (Papadopoulos and Saayman 1989).

Karen was referred to me, in my capacity as clinical psychologist/family therapist in the British National Health Service, by her family medical general practitioner, who asked me to treat her "AIDS phobia." She was approaching sixteen, and she was attending a prestigious church school where she was an excellent pupil. Her parents were in a panic because Karen, without any apparent reason, began to be afraid that she would "catch AIDS." As a result, she was washing her hands excessively—to a degree that the skin was peeling off them.

I asked to meet with her whole family, as usual explaining that I like to get as full a picture of the problem as possible. She was brought by her parents: her father was about 65, a softly spoken engineer; and her mother was in her middle 50's, an energetic woman who a few years earlier had changed career and moved from teaching to becoming a stockbroker. The problem was concrete and needed urgent attention. The mother was asking for direct practical advice and the father seemed desperate. Karen was a bit stunned by the whole affair and did not know how to understand what was going on. Rationally, she knew that there was no reason for concern (i.e., she neither had had any kind of sexual experience nor had she been exposed to any other infectious situations); yet, she was scared and bewildered.

Keeping my focus on their direct concerns about the symptom, I explored the broader family context in terms of how they perceived the problem and what effect they felt it had on them. Karen was the only child, and her parents had several siblings who were rather distant. The family was fairly isolated and each member was leading a rather self-contained life pursuing his or her career. It gradually emerged that both father and daughter were about to go through radical changes in their lives. The father was retiring in a few months' time, and at about the same time Karen was finishing school. Remarkably, the father did not know exactly what he was going to do after retirement and, similarly, Karen had several ideas but no concrete plans about what she would do after her graduation. It seemed to me that all three were finding it difficult to contemplate the substantial changes about to occur to the whole family.

I felt a great deal of affection for all of them and they seemed to have corresponding feelings towards me. I found them most likeable, and realized that the feelings and particular kind of care I caught myself having for them had the warmth of a grandfather's concern. The first couple of sessions went smoothly, and they all went along with me in examining the way they connected with the tragic symptom. In the meantime, their emphasis on the symptom diminished and they all seemed extremely eager to experience their newly found ability to communicate with each other. During all this time I was troubled by the violent nature of the symptom. I could understand that it referred to changes that were imminent in the family. However, the symptom referred to a violent type of change with life-threatening consequences. While being preoccupied with these ideas, I discovered that fifteen years earlier the father had had a mild heart attack, which they had completely forgotten about. When I used this information and said that they must be, somehow, concerned about the father's health after the retirement, they all—much to my surprise—had tears in their eyes.

In the subsequent sessions, we talked about the opportunity that the symptom offered them to get together as a family before the big changes of the father's retirement and Karen's possible leaving home, and to interrelate in ways which they had never done before. They were extremely engaged, and their attention to the symptom was constantly diminishing. At the end of the sessions, mother would invariably say something like, "By the way, Karen seems to be washing her hands less now."

About a month before Karen's graduation, my secretary told me that the family had phoned to cancel the session because the father had died suddenly. He had had a massive heart attack. The reader can imagine the shock I felt at hearing the news. However, I was also filled with awe. Our work does, indeed, touch the mysteries of life and death. Several weeks later, I received a moving letter from the mother thanking me for the opportunity I offered them to "become a real family" before her husband's death. She also mentioned that Karen had stopped her compulsive hand-washing.

There are many observations one could make about this case. Perhaps the most important one would be about the methodology: any causal approach would lead to nonsensical conclusions. Therapy did not cause father's death, neither did his heart illness cause Karen's symptom. All of these events, as well as the images and feelings experienced by all of us (therapist and family), were connected indeed; but not in a reductive and causal manner. Jung would have called it "synchronistic," and systemic family therapists "systemic." Perhaps they are talking about the same thing, but from different perspectives.

A different therapeutic approach could have focused on the sexual overtones in the relationship between Karen and her father. Obviously, there were definitely sexual conflicts unresolved within Karen, as well as Oedipal themes in connection with all three of them. Another approach could have concentrated on the transactions among them in order to find more appropriate ways of communicating. AFT enabled us to utilize the interactional aspects of the network of archetypal images in ways that facilitated family as well as individual shifts. The meaning of the symptom was appreciated in its imagistic and interactional dimensions.

I almost feel the need to apologize for the dramatic nature of this clinical example. Obviously, not all therapeutic work has such a startling outcome. However, this vignette seems to create an impact which would enable the reader to relate more directly with the material presented above. Therefore, any further detailed discussion, isolating specific processes for didactic purposes, would appear superfluous.

Summary

As might have become apparent, the central premises of AFT are also the points where Jung's analytical psychology and modern systemic family therapy converge; these are all interconnected and it is difficult to isolate them. However, they may be summed up as follows:

The Meaning of the Symptom

The symptom is not a meaningless result of an accidental misfortune and, therefore, the emphasis of therapy cannot possibly be its removal at all cost. The symptom has a meaning not only for the person who carries it but also for her or his family. By placing it in its broader collective/systemic, and imagistic/narrative contexts, we may be able to connect with its meaning as well as, possibly, its purpose.

Therapist's Position

The therapist is not an external objective observer who offers his or her expertise in a detached, technological manner. The therapist is part of the system and therefore has no choice but to access her or his own human responses to the situation. Jung's alchemical metaphor of therapy and the image of the wounded healer are just two examples of this awareness.

Self and Others

Individualistic or exclusively intrapsychic approaches to problems are insufficient. The individual in both Jungian and systemic approaches is not an isolated entity; that individual is defined in terms of the others and of broader structures which contain both the self and the other. Thus the self and the other are not only in constant interaction with themselves, but also with the various Collective Structures of Meaning (archetypes, images, ideological and social systems, etc.). Therefore, patient and therapist can only work meaningfully if they can locate themselves in broader systemic contexts within which they are contained. This means that therapy is a multidimensional activity, including intrapsychic, interpersonal, socio-cultural, imagistic, ecological, political, and other perspectives.

Methodology

To be able to move freely among these contexts, the therapist will need to abandon any one-sided methodologies such as reductive, causal, and linear approaches. Both Jung and family therapists have attacked such one-dimensional methodologies and have attempted to articulate alternatives to them: Jung put forward the ideas of "synchronicity," the "and/and rather than either/or" method, and the "union of opposites," to name but a few; and systemic family therapists have written about "circular," "systemic," "non-linear" epistemologies.

Archetypal and Systemic Structures

Both structures refer to broader wholes within which individuals interrelate. The interactional dimension of the archetype and the intrapsychic dimension of the system seem to have been neglected or under-emphasized. AFT attempts to reconnect the two in a way in which they may both benefit from each other. The ideas about Collective Structures of Meaning, and Network of Archetypal Images seem to be fruitful in conveying the best of both worlds within a coherent new theoretical structure with direct clinical applicability.

Epilogue

In an article in 1985 appropriately entitled "Extending the family (from entanglement to embrace)," James Hillman justifiably attacked the prevailing myth in the Western world according to which family is perceived as a restricting cage for the individual. The same myth "insists that ego is strengthened and full personality achieved away from familial ties and pressures" (7). Hillman accused sociological, psychoanalytic, and developmental theorists for this distorted view of family. Yet, he does not assign any responsibility to analytical psychologists for implicitly or explicitly supporting and even fueling such a myth with their own misunderstood suspicions of the collective. However, he seems to take it upon himself to demonstrate that a proper approach to analytical psychology cannot condone such a myth. The gist of his article was therefore "to turn the vice of entrapment in the personal family into an archetypal recognition of family as the supreme metaphor for sustaining the human condition" (6).

A parallel attempt to rehabilitate the family within analytical psychology was undertaken by Papadopoulos in his paper on "Adolescents and Homecoming" (1987). Within a different framework from that of Hillman, Papadopoulos argued for the extension of the notion of "homecoming" beyond its narrow literary and regressive meaning, and for the inclusion in it of more positive teleological and systemic potential. Central to that argument was a reading of "*The Odyssey*" according to which Odysseus' homecoming quest was not seen as an individualist "heroic" adventure, but was appreciated within the context of re-establishing Odysseus' meaningful relationships within the network of his own nuclear, extended, as well as "archetypal" families.

The intention of this chapter, in tune with these two articles, is not only to present a way of how a Jungian approach to working with families can be developed, but also to argue that an archetypal framework cannot possibly ignore the organizing systemic structures which interact at all levels with what is perceived as the intrapsychic world of the individual. This means that broader systemic considerations are endemic to any archetypal approach and thus the family in its full imagistic panoply cannot possibly be overlooked. Moreover, it is important to emphasize that the similarities between an archetypal approach and modern systemic family therapy approaches are not restricted to the actual content of their theories and practices but also include the very epistemology which informs them.

Ultimately, the content and epistemology of any therapeutic approach should be in harmony, closely informing one another. For example, when one approaches the family from a personal perspective, it is then appropriate to adopt a more linear, historical, and causal-reductive epistemology. Conversely, a therapist with an implicit or explicit causal-reductive epistemology would *perforce* approach the family from a personal perspective. This means that what would constitute evidence in that particular psychological work would be issues of historical causality. For example, emphasis would be given to the investigation of specific characteristics of parents and their own unresolved psychological conflicts. These would be accepted as causative of the individual patient's present predicament in a linear fashion. Inherent to this approach would be the assumption that the individual would need to free himself or herself from the "entrapment" of the family to achieve the ideal state of independence. However, if one were to adopt a more archetypal approach, the inherent epistemology would be more "circular" or synchronistic; and vice versa, a non-linear epistemology would dictate broader archetypal considerations. This would mean that the cause and effect would not be seen as sequential in a linear and causal fashion. As has been said by many authors in different ways and forms, it is not only the past that shapes the present, but also the present that shapes the past. This is so because one cannot possibly reify these concepts in a static mold. The past is not an undisputed set of historical "facts," but it depends on how the person defines it now. Thus, the patient's present predicament would not be accepted as a passive result of previous causes which could be investigated reductively from the individual's own history. Instead, it would be appreciated that the influence would be mutual and interactional, and thus circular. Moreover, both the individual and his or her family, insofar as they also belong to a broader organizing network, will also interact with those realms. These epistemological considerations are part and parcel of an archetypal approach and they constitute a common area with systemic family therapies.

Jung himself was acutely aware of the importance of the epistemological context that informs our therapeutic practices. In

1935, prompted by "the accusation . . . that the newer psychotherapy" (with which he identified) "is concerned too much with philosophical problems and not enough with the minutiae of case-histories" (par. 1042), he warned of the dangers of abandoning our epistemological vigilance:

> The empirical intellect, occupying itself with the minutiae of case-histories, involuntarily imports its own philosophical premises not only into the arrangement but also into the judgment of the material and even into the apparently objective presentation of data. (1935, par. 1042)

Further along, he observed that "a system of healing that fails to take account of the epoch making *representation collectives* of a political, economic, philosophical, or religious nature, or assiduously refuses to recognize them as actual forces, hardly deserves the name therapy" (par. 1043). These strong words reflect Jung's remarkably modern sensitivity to the importance of epistemological considerations in relation to our therapeutic practices. Yet, analytical psychologists after him were either reluctant or unable to follow that sensitivity. And we are faced today with the situation that it is mainly systemic family therapists who continue along the Jungian epistemological directions. Perhaps the old accusation that Jungian analysts are too "philosophical" and not sufficiently "clinical" has not lost its crippling venom, after all!

Note

This chapter is a substantially revised version of the article: "Towards a Jungian Approach to Family Therapy," written by Renos Papadopoulos and Graham Saayman, and published in Harvest: Journal for Jungian Studies 35 (1989): 95–120.

References

Aristotelis. 1965. *De Arte Poetica Liber*. Ed. Rudolf Kassel. Oxford: Clarendon Press.

Bateson, G. 1973. The cybernetics of "self": a theory of alcoholism. In *Steps to an Ecology of Mind.* St. Albans: Paladin. 280–308.

Bernstein, J. 1992. Beyond the personal: analytical psychology applied to groups and nations. In *C. G. Jung: Critical Assessments*. Ed. R. K. Papadopoulos. Vol. 4. London: Routledge. 22–37.

Boyd, R. D., ed. 1991. *Personal Transformations in Small Groups. A Jungian Perspective*. London: Routledge.

Bührmann, M. V. 1981. Xhentsa and Inthlombe: a Xhosa healing ritual. *Journal of Analytical Psychology* 26: 187–201.

———. 1984. Tentative views on dream therapy by Xhosa diviners. In *Jung in Modern Perspective* Ed. by R. K. Papadopoulos and G. S. Saayman. London: Wildwood House. 135–51.

Cronen, V. E. and Pearce, W. B. 1985. Towards an explanation of how the Milan method works: an invitation to a systemic epistemology and the evolution of family systems. In *Applications of Systemic Family Therapy*. Ed. D. Campbell and R. Draper. London: Grune and Stratton. 69–84.

Cunningham, A. and Saayman, G. S. 1984. Effective functioning in dual-career families: an investigation. *Journal of Family Therapy* 6: 365–80.

Epstein, N. B. and Bishop, D. S. 1981. Problem-centered systems therapy of the family. In *Handbook of Family Therapy*. Ed. S. Gurman and D. P. Kniskern. New York: Brunner/Mazel. 444–82.

Faber, P. A. 1990. Archetypal symbolism and the ideology of apartheid. In *Jung in the Context of Southern Africa*. Ed. G. S. Saayman. Boston: Sigo Press.

Faber, P. , Saayman, G. S., and Papadopoulos, R. K. 1983. Induced waking fantasy: its effects upon the archetypal content of nocturnal dreams. *Journal of Analytical Psychology* 28: 141–64.

Freud, S. 1914. Observations on transference-love. In S. E. 12: 159–71. London: Hogarth Press, 1958.

Guggenbühl-Craig, A. 1981. *Marriage: Dead or Alive*. Dallas: Spring Publications.

Hillman, J. 1985. Extending the family (from entanglement to embrace). *Texas Humanist* (March–April 1985): 6–11.

Jung, C. G. 1909. The family constellation. In *CW* 2: 466–79. London: Routledge and Kegan Paul, 1973.

———. 1910. A contribution to the psychology of rumour. In *CW* 4: 35–47. London: Routledge and Kegan Paul, 1973.

———. 1916. General aspects of dream psychology. In *CW* 8: 237–80. London: Routledge and Kegan Paul, 1969.

——. 1927. Women in Europe. In *CW* 10: 113–33. London: Routledge and Kegan Paul, 1970.

——. 1931. Marriage as a psychological relationship. In *CW* 17: 187–201. London: Routledge and Kegan Paul, 1970.

——. 1935. Editorial. For *Zentralblatt* 8.1. In *CW* 10: 547–51. London: Routledge and Kegan Paul, 1970.

——. 1945. After the catastrophe. In *CW* 10: 194–217. London: Routledge and Kegan Paul, 1970.

——. 1946a. The fight with the shadow. In *CW* 10: 218–26. London: Routledge and Kegan Paul, 1970.

——. 1946b. The psychology of the transference. In *CW* 16: 165–323. London: Routledge and Kegan Paul, 1966.

——. 1952. Synchronicity: an acausal connecting principle. In *CW* 8: 417–531. London: Routledge and Kegan Paul, 1969.

——. 1954a. Psychological aspects of the mother archetype. In *CW* 9 (Part I): 75–110. London: Routledge and Kegan Paul, 1968.

——. 1954b. On the nature of the psyche. In *CW* 8: 159–234. London: Routledge and Kegan Paul, 1969.

Jung, C. G. 1963. *Memories, Dreams, Reflections*. London: Random House.

Kaplan, J., Saayman, G. S. and Faber, P. A. 1981. An investigation of the use of nocturnal dream reports as diagnostic indices in the assessment of family problem solving. *Journal of Family Therapy* 3: 227–42.

Keeney, B. P. 1983. *Aesthetics of Change*. London: Guilford Press.

Lacan, J. 1968. *The Language of the Self.* Tr. A. Wilden. Baltimore: John Hopkins University Press.

——. 1977a. *The Four Fundamental Concepts of Psychoanalysis*. Tr. A. Sheridan. London: Hogarth.

——. 1977b. *Ecrits: A Selection*. Tr. A. Sheridan. London: Tavistock.

Lieberman, S. 1979. *Transgeneraticiational Family Therapy*. London: Croom Helm.

Mattoon, M. A. 1978. *Applied Dream Analysis: A Jungian Approach*. New York: Wiley.

Mindell, A. 1987. *The Dreambody in Relationships*. London: Routledge & Kegan Paul.

Newman, K. D. 1980. Counter-transference and consciousness. *Spring* 117–27.

Odajnyk, V. W. 1976. *Jung and Politics*. New York: Harper and Row.

Papadopoulos, R. K. 1980. The dialectic of the other in the psychology of C. G. Jung: a metatheoretical investigation. Ph.D. thesis. Cape Town, South Africa: University of Cape Town.

_____. 1984. Jung and the concept of the other. In *Jung in Modern Perspective*. Ed. R. K. Papadopoulos and G. S. Saayman. London: Wildwood House. 54–88.

_____. 1987. *Adolescents and Homecoming*. London: Guild of Pastoral Psychology.

_____, ed. 1992. *C. G. Jung: Critical Assessments*. In 4 vols. London: Routledge.

_____. 1994. "Wotan's wrath: Jungian reflections on experiences of working with Bosnian ex-camp prisoners." Lecture delivered at the Association of Jungian Analysts.

_____. and Saayman, G. 1989. Towards a Jungian approach to family therapy. *Harvest: Journal for Jungian Studies* 35: 95–120.

Plaut. A. 1974. The transference in analytical psychology. In *Technique in Jungian Analysis*. Ed. M. Fordham, R. Gordon, J. Hubback and K. Lambert. London: Heinemann, 152–60.

———. 1993. *Analysis Analysed. When the Map becomes the Territory*. London: Routledge.

Progoff, I. 1969. *Jung's Psychology and Its Social Meaning*. New York: Julian Press.

Rychlak, J. F. 1981. *Personality and Psychotherapy*. Boston: Houghton Mifflin.

———. 1984. Jung as dialectician and teleologist. In *Jung in Modern Perspective*. Ed. R. K. Papadopoulos and G. S. Saayman. London: Wildwood House, 34–53.

Saayman, G. S., Faber, P. A., and Saayman, R. V. 1988. Archetypal factors revealed in the study of marital breakdown: a Jungian perspective. *Journal of Analytical Psychology* 33: 253–76.

Samuels, A. 1985. *Jung and the Post-Jungians*. London: Routledge & Kegan Paul.

———. 1993. *The Political Psyche*. London: Routledge.

Selvini-Palazzoli, M., Boscolo, L., Cecchin, G. and Prata, G. 1980. 1978. *Paradox and Counterparadox*. New York: Jason Aronson.

———. Hypothesizing-circularity-neutrality: three guidelines for the conductor of the session. *Family Process* 19: 3–12.

Shands, H. C. 1971. *The War with Words*. Paris: Mouton.

Shuttleworth-Jordan, A., Saayman, G. S., and Faber, P. A. 1988. A systematised method for dream analysis in a group setting. *International Journal of Group Psychotherapy* 38: 473–89.

Spiegelman, J. M. 1980. The image of the Jungian analyst and the problem of authority. *Spring* 101–16.

Stevens, A. 1982. *Archetype: A Natural History of the Self.* London: Routledge and Kegan Paul.

———. 1986. *Witheymead: A Jungian Community for the Healing Arts.* London: Coventure.

Strubel, R. 1980. Individuation and group. In *Proceedings of the Eighth International Congress for Analytical Psychology.* Ed. J. Beebe. Fellbach-Oeffngen: Bonz, 1983. 287–97.

Vetere, A. 1987. General system theory and the family: a critical evaluation. In *Ecological Studies of Family Life.* Ed. A. Vetere and A. Gale. New York: John Wiley, 18–33.

Watzslawick, P., Beavin, J., and Jackson, D. 1967. *Pragmatics of Human Communication.* New York: W. W. Norton.

Young-Eisendrath, P. 1984. *Hags and Heroes: A Feminist Approach to Jungian Psychotherapy with Couples.* Toronto: Inner City Books.

Zinkin, L. 1994. The dialogical principle in group analysis and analytical psychology. Harvest: *Journal for Jungian Studies* 40: 7–24.

***Dr. Renos Papadopoulos** is a training Jungian analyst and family therapist who lectures widely in England and abroad; he is the editor of "Harvest: Journal for Jungian Studies," and of the "Newsletter of the International Journal for Analytical Psychology." Dr. Papadopoulos holds appointments as Consultant Clinical Psychologist at the Tavistock Clinic, London, and as Professor of Analytical Psychology at the Centre for Psychoanalytic Studies of the University of Essex. His last book is a four-volume edited collection of essays entitled "C.G. Jung: Critical Assessments." Dr. Papadopoulos has worked with victims in Chernobyl, Soweto, and Slovenia, and, more recently, with former prisoners from the Bosnian camps evacuated to the U.K. by the Red Cross.*

Made in United States
Orlando, FL
04 November 2026

90201204R00104